# The
# Attachment
# Pregnancy

# The
# Attachment
# Pregnancy

### The ULTIMATE GUIDE to
## *Bonding with Your Baby*

Your Early
Start to
*Attachment
Parenting*

**Laurel Wilson** IBCLC, CCCE, CLD, CLE *and*
**Tracy Wilson Peters** CCCE, CLD, CLE

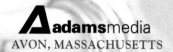

AVON, MASSACHUSETTS

ISBN 10: 1-4405-7010-8
ISBN 13: 978-1-4405-7010-0
eISBN 10: 1-4405-7011-6
eISBN 13: 978-1-4405-7011-7

Printed in the United States of America.

10  9  8  7  6  5  4  3  2  1

Published by Adams Media, a division of F+W Media, Inc.
57 Littlefield Street, Avon, MA 02322. U.S.A.
www.adamsmedia.com

**Library of Congress Cataloging-in-Publication Data**
Wilson, Laurel, author.
    The attachment pregnancy / Laurel Wilson, IBCLC, CCCE, CLD, CLE and Tracy Wilson Peters, CCCE, CLD, CLE.
        pages cm
    Includes bibliographical references and index.
    ISBN-13: 978-1-4405-7010-0 (pbk.)
    ISBN-10: 1-4405-7010-8 (pbk.)
    ISBN-13: 978-1-4405-7011-7 (ebook)
    ISBN-10: 1-4405-7011-6 (ebook)
    1. Pregnancy. 2. Pregnancy--Psychological aspects. 3. Motherhood--Psychological aspects.
    4. Mother and child. I. Peters, Tracy Wilson, author. II. Title.
    RG556.W55 2014
    618.2--dc23
                        2013034540

This publication is designed to provide accurate and authoritative information with regard to the subject matter covered. It is sold with the understanding that the publisher is not engaged in rendering legal, accounting, or other professional advice. If legal advice or other expert assistance is required, the services of a competent professional person should be sought.

—From a *Declaration of Principles* jointly adopted by a Committee of the American Bar Association and a Committee of Publishers and Associations

This book is intended as general information only, and should not be used to diagnose or treat any health condition. In light of the complex, individual, and specific nature of health problems, this book is not intended to replace professional medical advice. The ideas, procedures, and suggestions in this book are intended to supplement, not replace, the advice of a trained medical professional. Consult your physician before adopting any of the suggestions in this book, as well as about any condition that may require diagnosis or medical attention. The author and publisher disclaim any liability arising directly or indirectly from the use of this book.

Many of the designations used by manufacturers and sellers to distinguish their product are claimed as trademarks. Where those designations appear in this book and F+W Media was aware of a trademark claim, the designations have been printed with initial capital letters.

Cover image © iStockphoto.com/katalinamas.

*This book is available at quantity discounts for bulk purchases.*
*For information, please call 1-800-289-0963.*

# DEDICATION

Without you both, Trevor and Ryan, the seed would never have been planted. Without you, Danny, the flower would never have bloomed. This book is for you, the most generous and loving of men.

—Laurel Wilson

This book is dedicated to my husband and best friend, Mark Peters. Mark has been my biggest fan and greatest source of support for more than two decades and there is no question that without his love and support this book would not be possible. Thank you, Mark, for working through your lunch hours and vacations so that I could realize my dreams. To my children, Hunter and Foster, who shared their mama with many families while they were growing up and still proudly support the work that I do. You are both my greatest teachers and my greatest inspiration, and I am very honored to be your mother; I love you both more than a dedication could ever say.

—Tracy Wilson Peters

# Contents

# Foreword

What happens when science meets love, and for the first time the two are in perfect agreement? The result is a book such as *The Attachment Pregnancy* by pregnancy experts Tracy Wilson Peters and Laurel Wilson. In a style that is full of warmth and straight-talk, this book brings mothers the most revolutionary scientific discoveries about the transformative power of their maternal love. Readers will be amazed to learn how a mother's love literally grows the child's brain and regulates their heart rhythms—in the womb, through labor, and afterwards. Only a pair of experienced and loving mothers and childbirth professionals—like Tracy and Laurel—can speak with the voice of wisdom mixed with genuine affection for parents and their babies. They tell the story from the inside. They talk the talk because they have walked the walk; there is not a patronizing word to be found in these pages.

Tracy and Laurel have rolled up their sleeves and filled this book with tons of practical help for expectant and new mothers. There are plenty of enjoyable activities for taking care of the body, mind, and spirit, with a special focus on this most important element: creating, maintaining, and surrounding oneself with emotionally supportive relationships to encourage the deep bond between mother and child. At every turn, the practical advice offered rests on the concrete footings of leading-edge science and the best knowledge gathered by two highly experienced practitioners.

In twenty-five years as a psychologist in private practice, I have lost count of the mothers I have spoken with who have felt utterly disempowered by their care during pregnancy. The rewards of a sensitively ushered pregnancy can be blissful and delicious, while securing a lifetime of psychological strength and health for the baby. A revolution is warranted in how we conceive of pregnancy and childbirth: with love and attention rather than fear. This wonderful book is a clarion call to bring the maternal back to maternity.

It is the aim of this book to put the mother in the driver's seat, with all the support she needs at her fingertips to encourage attachment between mother and baby. Mothers will feel uplifted, the importance of their role valued and elevated. The extensive and simply explained information in these pages helps you to explore your feelings to know what is best for you and your baby.

Your baby is a conscious person with a thinking mind, the full range of human emotion, and the capacity to be in deep connection with you well before birth—this is an awe-inspiring discovery! In these pages you will be shown how to consciously communicate with your unborn child, and how to remain deeply attuned to yourself and your baby throughout pregnancy, labor, and the sublime moments of bonding that follow. You will be surprised to learn how much is known today about your unborn and newborn baby's intelligence and capacity for relationship. The most exciting news is that as you meet your baby's needs for connection, pleasure, love, and affection, you literally change his or her brain chemistry and neurobiology, preparing your child for a lifetime of security, success, and psychological wellness. This idea is no longer the stuff of sentimentality; it is underpinned by modern brain science and mother–infant attachment research. Beautiful descriptions along the way make the book a pleasure to read and help to ground the information in your mind. For too long, parents have been spooked by ideas about pregnancy that range from the distressing to the terrifying. How can anyone relax, let go, and trust the pregnancy process after a lifetime's exposure to frightful imagery? It is now clear that many complications during pregnancy can be eliminated when mothers are empowered, reassured, and supported by people who are trusted and familiar and with whom they feel safe. When emotional needs are met, medical wellness and attachment pregnancy is far more likely to follow. The mission these two authors have valiantly undertaken is to return this maternal and natural right to mothers. What has been taken away is now given back. The rewards of a lovingly supported pregnancy are for life; they ripple into every area of human endeavor, health, and social functioning—for babies as for their parents. Long may Tracy and Laurel shout their message from the rooftops!

For the delicate and intimate attachment pregnancy, this book offers a unique recipe. It is a recipe for an elixir of "falling in love"; the foundation for a most wonderful start to a growing family's life together—and the best thing is, the authors' suggestions are endorsed by the best of modern science. The miracle of this primal bond is encoded as a program; it is neurologically hardwired in the brains of both mother and baby. Tracy and Laurel take you by the hand and show you, one step at a time. They are two warmhearted and wise mothers walking you through the most profound experience of your life. Therein lie the secrets to a pleasurable and joyous pregnancy, parenting, a calmer baby, healthy brain development, and a lifetime of psychological wellness for your child. Mothers: read on, and with Tracy and Laurel's guidance, take back what has always been rightfully yours. By showing the way to a far more peaceful, loving, and emotionally attached pregnancy, this book has the potential to change the world. It is my deepest wish that it be read by millions.

—Robin Grille, Psychologist, Parent Educator, and Author of *Parenting for a Peaceful World* and *Heart to Heart Parenting*

# Introduction

At no other time during life can a mother and her baby possibly be more connected than during pregnancy. During this period of primal attachment, you and your child are physically connected by the umbilical cord and the placenta, and you are also emotionally connected as a result of the molecular messages being exchanged along this pathway. But how can you use this connection to form an even closer bond to your unborn baby? How can you ensure that this closeness you and your baby share will continue after the baby is born? Attachment pregnancy gives you the tools you need to forge a bond with your baby that can never be broken.

Babies are conscious and aware in utero, and their experience in the womb forms the foundation for the rest of their life. You are not just a vessel carrying a baby. You are your child's world; the environment that you provide for your baby with your body, thoughts, and feelings determines how he or she will develop. This extraordinary period of development creates something called *the motherbaby bond*, where every thought, emotion, and feeling that you experience is shared and incorporated into the development of your baby. In fact, at no other time in your child's life does the motherbaby bond have the power to influence who your child will be, both emotionally and physically, than during pregnancy and the first years of his or her life. Fortunately, the advice, activities, and information found within *The Attachment Pregnancy* will help you connect with your baby during each trimester, creating a deeper intimacy, awareness, and profound attachment between the two of you.

Throughout the book, the unique and groundbreaking concepts found in each part focus on one developmental period and essential concept of attachment pregnancy that will help you build and then strengthen the motherbaby bond. This BOND is formed by:

- **B**e-ing, which focuses in on the beginning of your journey toward motherhood and attachment
- **O**bserving, which focuses on the first trimester where you need to learn to become mindful and observant of yourself and your baby
- **N**ourishing, which focuses on the second trimester where you need to learn to love, nourish, and care for yourself, your baby, and your relationships
- **D**eciding, which focuses on the third trimester and beyond and helps you think about and prepare for giving birth and life with your new baby

Together these concepts are designed to help you truly experience an attachment pregnancy.

If you are thinking about conceiving a child or trying to conceive, now is the time to do the personal work that will enable you to embrace your pregnancy, attach to your baby, and prepare for parenthood. You have a unique opportunity here and now to become the parent you want to be. And if you are already pregnant, you can use the advice found throughout to transform your life and the life of your baby through Conscious Attachment and Agreement, to set your intentions for your pregnancy and parenting to design a life that will support a healthy bond between you and your baby, and to create a secure attachment between you and your baby from the very beginning.

Attachment pregnancy starts on an emotional level the moment you become mindful of your baby as a person; as an expectant mother, you have the ability to decide what you want your pregnancy to look like and even more important, what you want your experience to feel like. What you expect becomes what you think about. What you think about becomes what you experience. What you experience becomes a reality for you and your newborn. You and your baby should experience the love and connection that attachment pregnancy offers, so start to make the changes that are right for your family from this moment forward. Enjoy the journey!

# PART 1

# Be-ing: The Beginning

## **B** O N D

### **B** stands for Be-ing

> "What lies before us and what lies behind us is but a small matter compared to what lies within us."
>
> –RALPH WALDO EMERSON, Poet and Author

In the beginning there was only you, and then in a flash, you became two. You are now intimately connected to another human being that you are responsible for. All of a sudden your life, your thoughts, your relationships, and your attitudes have a greater reach than your private world.

How you live your life and, just as important, how you *feel* about your life, actually shape every cell, every organ, and the very personality of your child. This part of *The Attachment Pregnancy*, which is about Be-ing, helps you understand how your thoughts and feelings can impact your pregnancy and either magnify or minimize the bond that you have with your baby. Here you'll learn that your ability to be conscious and aware of your world is the foundation for an attachment pregnancy. In this part you will discover that you can begin to develop a conscious connection to your baby simply by becoming more aware of your surroundings, your relationships, and most importantly, your baby. Read on . . .

# CHAPTER 1

# What Is Be-ing?

> "Before you were conceived I wanted you. Before you were born I loved you. Before you were here an hour I would die for you. This is the miracle of life."
>
> ~Maureen Hawkins, Author

You have the opportunity to manifest the pregnancy you want with every thought you think, feeling you feel, and action you take. Be-ing is a state of consciousness that allows your attachment pregnancy to come to light. The literal definition of consciousness is the state of being awake and aware of one's surroundings. What does "awake and aware" really mean? The definition of consciousness for an attachment pregnancy is the act of being fully aware and fully present in your thoughts, feelings, and actions. It means being in a state of mindfulness, where you are observing the world around you. You are tuned in to your thoughts and feelings, but not necessarily allowing them to drive your actions. When you choose to become conscious during pregnancy, you are choosing an attachment pregnancy. You are choosing the ultimate motherbaby bond.

Becoming conscious, or mindful, allows you to explore your relationship with yourself. Your positive relationship to "you" is the foundation for having a happy child, a happy family, and a happy life. You are important. You are literally the world in which your baby will be formed. Learning how to move into a state of Be-ing, or consciousness, will have a profound effect on your life and your family. When you become more aware and mindful of yourself, your life, your attitude, and your relationships, you can become more centered. This centering allows you to connect deep within to discover what is most important to you and your baby. Be-ing is the very foundation for the most important relationship of all: the relationship between you and your source. Your source is how you define your reason for being here, as well as how you define your relationship with everything in your world. This is different for every individual, whether you believe in God, a higher power, or simply that you have a unique purpose for being here in this life. Pregnancy is a time of deep reflection, a time to look at who you have been, who you are, and who you want to be. You will experience a shift; your life, as you know it, will change as you become a better "you" for your baby. The journey of attachment pregnancy will transform you.

## Conscious or Subconscious?

What is the difference between being in a conscious state of Be-ing and being in a state of subconscious awareness? Scientists have found that most people's subconscious minds dictate their daily actions more than 90 percent of the time. This means that, for the most part, you are not paying attention to what is happening in you and around you. For example, how many times have you driven your car down a familiar road, toward a familiar destination, and realized as you arrived that you have no recollection of how you got there? That is because your subconscious mind has memorized the details and past events of your life. Your subconscious mind allows you to operate on autopilot most of the time. Autopilot isn't *always* a bad thing.

Autopilot has an important role; it allows you to function without having to use up too much brain power to simply get through the day. You don't have to spend too much energy figuring out the best way to get dressed, or to make your breakfast, or to interact with the familiar people in your life. Your subconscious mind helps you move through the world in a safe and comfortable manner. This allows your conscious mind to have more energy to process new experiences. The problem is that your subconscious mind starts to create habits out of everything you do. As time goes by, you become less and less likely to fully experience anything new. You are a creature of habit. It's your very nature.

These habits create an illusion of safety all around you. You react to life's events according to all of the memories your subconscious mind has stored, whether these memories are in your best interest or not. For example, if you had a frightening experience with a dog as a child, your mind may have stored the memory that dogs are dangerous, and your subconscious mind creates ways for you to avoid dogs and to react as though any dog you see is a threat. Your mind is protecting you based on your past experience, even if it's not necessarily accurate. Is every dog a threat? No, but your subconscious mind might think it is. The mere act of living causes most of us to become less conscious, as we operate more and more on autopilot as we age. So what is a mother to do?

## Make a Conscious Choice

Be-ing is actually a choice that you will make in every moment of your pregnancy. When you move into a state of consciousness, you become aware of everything around you. You become tuned in to your thoughts and your feelings. This is called being *mindful*. The more tuned in you become, the more you begin to realize that the thoughts and feelings you experience may not be an accurate portrayal of the present moment. Instead, these thoughts and feelings are a direct reflection of your past experiences. After all, it's human nature to constantly apply your history to your present, like watching a TV show over and over again. You cannot change the TV show until you are aware that you have been watching the same program over and over and want to change the channel. This realization is the first step to Be-ing.

When you practice Be-ing, you take the time to listen to your thoughts and ask yourself: Where did that thought come from? How does it make me feel? How is it affecting my baby? Is my current emotional state causing these thoughts? Is my reaction realistic based on what is actually happening, or is it related to something I experienced in my past?

Once you realize that a thought is not "real" or is not beneficial for you or your baby, you have the power to change your mind and change your reactions to various situations for the better. After all, your feelings are shared with your baby, and the more you can positively shape your thoughts and feelings, the more you will experience the motherbaby bond. As you become aware of the power of your thoughts and how they affect your baby, it becomes easier to create an attachment pregnancy. Why? Because when you're actively thinking about how your thoughts, feelings, and reactions affect your child, you will become motivated to make positive changes that will benefit both you and your baby.

> "Making the decision to have a child—it is momentous. It is to decide forever to have your heart go walking around outside your body."
>
> ~Elizabeth Stone, Author of *A Boy I Once Knew*

## What if You Don't Practice Be-ing?

When you don't practice consciousness during pregnancy, you remain unaware of your behavior, actions, thoughts, and habits. You also remain unaware of how these behaviors, actions, thoughts, and habits affect your baby. This state of unconsciousness limits your ability to create change during your pregnancy and be fully present. If you do not practice Be-ing, you aren't aware of what needs to change for you to experience a healthy and attached pregnancy. Each new day and each new relationship you develop presents opportunities to create positive change during pregnancy and a deeper motherbaby bond. You want to grab onto these opportunities with both hands in order to ensure a strong attachment pregnancy and a healthy, long-lasting relationship with your baby.

## Consciousness and Attachment

Old ideas have led us to believe that babies are solely at the mercy of their genes and biology. It was believed that pregnancy was based on biology, and children were the products of their parents' DNA. Emerging science has discovered that, while traditional biology does indeed have a role to play in the development of babies, it is not the only thing that matters. While every child will have a specific genetic blueprint, known as DNA, research has found that the internal environment (your thoughts, feelings, and beliefs) and external environment (food you eat, air you breathe, chemicals you are exposed to, etc.) can actually change the reading of your baby's blueprint during your pregnancy. It turns out that your choices affect the way your baby's body and mind will grow. You are a baby builder—how exciting!

Here is an example: Pregnancy and your growing baby are like the musicians and the instruments in an orchestra. Every orchestra has unique instruments and musicians, but you, the mother, are the conductor and the composer. You are writing your own symphony.

You choose the notes and the melody and, if there is something out of tune, you can change the music. You create the harmony. You are the maestro.

When you choose to conceive and grow your baby in a trusting, loving, peaceful state, she is formed in love. This process of choosing to be conscious and aware leads you to become an active participant in your life. What you think about, you bring about. Even if your baby's conception was a surprise, or if bringing your baby into the world at this time in your life seems challenging, you still have an opportunity to create an attachment pregnancy. When you choose to practice Be-ing during pregnancy, you directly impact the health and happiness of your child and strengthen the motherbaby bond.

If you are often unconscious of your reactions to people, events, and places, your body and your baby are still affected by those reactions. Unfortunately, many pregnant mothers live in a constant state of stress. When mothers allow their subconscious mind to be in control, instead of staying in a state of Be-ing, they create a cycle of chronic stress. When the body is chronically stressed, it constantly produces stress hormones, which negatively affect your pregnancy and your baby. In fact, chronic stress is one of the leading causes of illness in pregnancy, preterm delivery, and challenges with a newborn baby. Fortunately, once you become aware of this cycle, you have the ability to break it. You *can* learn how to manage stress during pregnancy by being more conscious of your life, taking control, and using stress-releasing techniques. Isn't it time to think about what you are thinking about?

# CHAPTER SUMMARY

Be-ing is the act of being conscious and aware of your surroundings. Through Be-ing, you learn how to become a nonjudgmental observer in your life, which strengthens the motherbaby bond and your attachment pregnancy. To participate in Be-ing, you must be fully aware and fully present in your thoughts, feelings, and actions. Remember:

- Your subconscious mind allows you to operate on autopilot most of the time. When you are in your subconscious mind, you forget to practice attachment pregnancy.

- The more aware you become, the more you begin to realize that the thoughts and feelings you are experiencing may not be an accurate portrayal of the present moment. Pay attention mindfully to your thoughts often.

- Your feelings are shared with your baby, and the more you can positively shape your thoughts and feelings, the more you will feel the motherbaby bond.

- Through the practice of Be-ing, you become aware of what needs to change for you to experience a healthy and attached pregnancy.

- Your choices and actions can affect the way your baby's body and mind will grow.

- During chronic stress, your body is constantly producing stress hormones, which can affect your pregnancy and your baby. Your awareness of this cycle of stress gives you the ability to break it and positively impact your attachment pregnancy.

# CHAPTER 2

# Positive Mental Attitudes

> **"The state of your life is nothing more than a reflection of the state of your mind."**
>
> ~Dr. Wayne Dyer, Motivational Speaker and Author

Is the glass half full or is the glass half empty? This question is one you have heard many times, but it is asked for a reason; it is central to an attachment pregnancy. How you answer that question affects your pregnancy and your baby, because it is a reflection of your mental attitude. Your mental attitude is your perception of your world, and this perception impacts your pregnancy and your baby. How you view your world determines your body's reaction to the world. Negative attitudes create stress in the body, and stress, as mentioned in Chapter 1, impacts every part of your pregnancy. It can, in fact, even impair your ability to truly feel attached to your baby. In this chapter, you'll learn how to view the glass as half full and how your positive mental attitude (PMA) can help strengthen your attachment pregnancy.

## Your World Is Your Baby's World

How many times have you heard yourself saying, "Life is just not fair," or "Why does this always happen to me?"

Sound familiar?

In every moment of your life you judge what is happening to you. Remember, your past experiences have preprogrammed your mind, and your thoughts reflect your memories instead of the reality of the present situation. Ask yourself if you are more likely to interpret situations as positive or negative. Unfortunately, negativity is all too familiar for most people, and it turns out that they may have actually been born that way. During pregnancy and early infancy, the emotional states and stress levels of the mother program a baby's subconscious, that part of the mind that influences one's thoughts and actions the majority of the time. Your subconscious thoughts (as opposed to your thoughts when you are Be-ing) are a direct result of how your brain developed in the womb and your first years of life, based on how your mother perceived the world.

Until now, it was believed that a baby's only connection to her mother was via the umbilical cord, which provides nutrients and blood to the baby. However, your baby is not living in a world separate from you; quite the opposite is true. Your baby's world *is* your world. You are intimately connected, sharing feelings, tastes, sounds, and chemical messages. Imagine yourself as a computer, filled with data, files, memory, and software. The baby can be seen as a flash drive, which connects for a short time to the computer to download all of the important data. Once all of the files have been copied and the flash drive (baby) is disconnected (born) from the computer (mother), the data on the flash drive remains for future use. Though the files can be altered, they are the foundation for everything.

## Clean Out Your Hard Drive

Unintentionally and unconsciously, your mother, based on her stress level and emotions, might have programmed your hard drive with messages that the world was a scary and dangerous place. Remember, you mother's reaction to her life was based on what she perceived as stressful. Her attitude toward her experiences during pregnancy and the early years of your life formed the foundation of who you are today.

Just as your mother's world-view shaped you, your world-view or attitude will form the foundation for your child's life. What programs or files are you storing on your internal hard drive? Are there files that you need to delete or alter; new programs to add while you grow your baby? What messages will you send to your baby? For the most part, the subconscious mind is programmed during conception through toddlerhood, and ultimately determines one's attitudes and perceptions of the world. This is because the part of the brain that is developed in utero is the thinking and feeling part of the brain. The emotional experiences your child has in the womb direct her brain development while the intellectual part of her brain matures. When a baby experiences chronic stress in utero, it physically changes how the limbic, or emotional, center of the brain develops. The brain develops according to the chemical messages it receives from the mother. A stressed mother creates a baby whose brain is wired for stress. On the other hand, a mother who manages her stress, and practices Be-ing, helps her baby's brain develop to manage stress as well. You will learn more about stress in pregnancy and your baby's brain in Chapter 7. If your baby has the opportunity to experience the world as a safe and loving place during pregnancy and the first years of life, she can develop a positive mental attitude and her mind will seek opportunity. She'll then see the world as a place to explore and enjoy. This is the foundation for positive parenting, which begins with an attachment pregnancy.

> "Your assumptions are your windows on the world. Scrub them off every once in a while, or the light won't come in."
> ~Alan Alda, Actor

## Have a Positive Mental Attitude

Having a positive mental attitude (PMA) does not come easily or naturally to most people because the subconscious mind is usually programmed for negativity. Developing a PMA during your pregnancy will not only change your life, but the life of your baby. It changes the experience of the situations from being annoying, stressful, or even tragic to opportunities for growth. Looking for the upside of a challenging situation or negative thought can turn "Why aren't there any parking places near my doctor's office?" into "My baby and I will benefit from this short walk to the office." When you focus your energy on seeing the good in life, you will see the good.

### Opportunity Knocks

The world is full of opportunities if you choose to find them. Opportunities are not just for a select, lucky few. Pregnancy is the perfect time to assess your perceptions and begin to adopt an attitude of gratitude and optimism. Optimistic people attract what they want. They attract good jobs, good friends, and good experiences; the things and circumstances in life that they want. Optimistic people attract positive things and circumstances because they are always on the lookout for them. If you believe that a good life is possible, opportunities will begin to manifest themselves. The pregnant optimist will attract the people, situations, and attitudes that are more likely to support a healthy and positive attachment pregnancy.

People who consciously practice gratitude report higher levels of alertness, enthusiasm, determination, optimism, and energy. They also experience less depression and stress and are more likely to feel loved. These are all important states for both you *and* your baby during pregnancy. The pregnant optimist is more likely to engage in healthy pregnancy behaviors (such as exercising and eliminating unhealthy habits), have a healthier immune system, and potentially experience less prenatal and postpartum depression. In addition, gratitude releases positive hormones, such as oxytocin (the love hormone) and beta-endorphins, which support a healthy pregnancy. These hormones help a mother and baby bond, reduce stress, and encourage a healthy mental attitude. In fact, studies have shown that the hormones related to optimistic thoughts work better than drugs on people who are clinically depressed. Your brain is a natural pharmacy, which can be used to your advantage during pregnancy, labor and delivery, and breastfeeding. Your body and mind are not separate, nor are your feelings separate from your baby's development.

## Are You an Optimist or a Pessimist?

Optimism is defined as a tendency to seek out, remember, and expect pleasurable experiences. Are you actively seeking happiness during your pregnancy? Are you expecting it? If your world-view does not support optimism, it is time to make some conscious changes. If you're not sure you're up to it, consider the child you are carrying. Do you want to raise a child who expects happiness and is confident and self-assured, or one who is fearful, anxious, and unhappy? Every mother wants to raise a happy child, and you're probably no exception. You can teach your child to love life, embrace change, and look for the good—even in unexpected situations—right from the start. Remember, you cannot shelter your baby from your experiences while you are pregnant. You are attached to your baby throughout pregnancy with every moment and every feeling and, while you may not be able to change what happens to you, you can change your attitude and reaction to your life. You are in control.

When you become aware of your perceptions, you can change them. You can choose whether to see a storm cloud or a cloud with a silver lining. It may take time and perspective to see the silver lining, but if you believe it is there, it will be. The things you at first perceive as negative can be the catalysts for a great change in your life. Having a PMA is really all about trusting yourself. When you trust yourself, you know that in any given situation, you have the power to choose how you feel about it. You can choose how or if you will react to it. Positive people know that even in the midst of chaos there lies unseen opportunity. When you look for opportunity, that's exactly what you'll find.

People with PMA know that they will be able to have just what they need when they need it. Teaching your child that she can trust that her needs will be met is a wonderful gift that you have the ability to give her. From the moment of conception, you have the incredible opportunity to be an optimistic, enthusiastic, loving mother, but how do you start?

## Baby Steps to Adopting a PMA

Developing a positive mental attitude will not happen just because you want it to. You must be willing to make some concrete steps to begin to literally change your mind. A commitment to positivity must be integrated into every part of your life. Being positive isn't something you try to do; it is something you become after consistent practice. This repetitive practice rewires your brain (and your baby's) from a negative perception to a positive one. The following information shows you how you can enhance your positivity practice during your attachment pregnancy and beyond.

## Use the Three Rs

The first step to adopting a PMA is recognizing negative thoughts when you have them. This requires active listening to your mind's self-talk. When you catch yourself thinking a negative thought, this is your opportunity to make a change. It is not easy to make this shift, nor will you always be aware of your subconscious mind controlling your actions, but every time you recognize a negative thought, it is an opportunity to become fully conscious. You have a chance to experience optimism *and* gratitude, and the key to embracing these and breaking the habit of negative thinking is to use the three Rs:

- **Recognize it:** Catch yourself thinking the negative thought and realize that this is actually a moment for mindfulness and awareness. Example: *I hate how my body looks during pregnancy.*
- **Review it:** Pause and consider the situation. Ask yourself, *Does this situation deserve my reaction, or am I reacting inappropriately? Is there another way I can look at this situation?* Example: *Why does my body look this way? I have extra weight due to my growing baby and body. This weight is necessary and helpful to my baby. This weight gain is only temporary and is a healthy sign of motherhood.*
- **Replace it:** Take a deep breath, focus on your heart and your baby, and consciously think a positive thought. Example: *I am grateful for my body's ability to sustain the life of my baby. I accept and love my growing body as a visible sign of the motherbaby bond.*

The more you practice using the three Rs, the more you will find yourself thinking positive thoughts in general. Consistently recognizing and changing your thoughts from negative to positive will become an integral part of your brain's hardwiring. Being positive will then simply become a part of your life.

ACTIVITY: PRACTICE THE THREE Rs

Take some time right now to practice the three Rs. Close your eyes and begin to pay attention to your thoughts. When a negative thought surfaces, begin to work through the steps and recognize, review, and replace it. When you have replaced the negative thought, take a few moments to experience this good feeling and the strong, loving attachment to your baby it fosters.

The more that you actively and consciously practice the power of positive thinking, the more it becomes second nature. Help yourself and your baby by creating reminders in your daily life to be positive. Place positive quotes on your desk at work, read positive books, and seek out positive people who will have a positive influence on you. Pay attention to what and who in your life makes you feel good . . . as well as what and who doesn't. You will learn more about creating boundaries with the people in your life in Chapter 5. ●

## Pregnancy Affirmations

Another way to increase your PMA during pregnancy is to practice using affirmations, positive statements of beliefs or truths that reflect your inner intentions. An example of a pregnancy affirmation is, "I am grateful for my pregnancy and healthy, growing baby." These statements affirm beliefs that your innermost being holds as true, even though at times your subconscious mind may be telling you that they are not. The repetition of writing affirmations, as well as saying them out loud, can help to change your subconscious mind when you believe the affirmations have the potential to be true. The more you repeat affirmations from a place of gratitude, the deeper they become rooted in your subconscious mind.

**34** The Attachment Pregnancy

However, if you're just repeating statements without believing them, you won't get the positive outcome you desire. The key to successful affirmations is practicing them while feeling the feeling that you will experience when the affirmations have manifested in your life. Stating affirmations to yourself while in a state of discouragement, irritation, or disbelief will not allow affirmations to change your mind. To receive the most benefit, you should imagine yourself as already experiencing the affirmation and resonate in that sensation for a bit before practicing your affirmations. Additionally, having your partner practice affirmations is a way that you can bond as a family and practice an attachment pregnancy together.

## ACTIVITY: PRACTICE AFFIRMATIONS

Read the following affirmations and select those that seem to speak to you. If you wish, write your own affirmations. Make a commitment to repeat these affirmations to yourself often throughout the day. Write them on your mirror, place them on your fridge, and hang them on your walls. Affirmations should always be stated in the present tense: "I am" versus "I will." They should be positive and start with the word "I" or "My." Affirmations that your partner can use are also provided below, because as you will learn later on in this book, developing a positive partner relationship will also benefit the motherbaby bond. The more that your partner practices affirmations about your pregnancy and your baby, the more positive he or she will feel as well. Remember to practice affirmations while in a state of gratitude.

### Affirmations for You
- My pregnant body is strong and capable.
- I am creating a happy, healthy, and loved baby.
- My body is healthy and I am happy.
- I accept that my pregnancy and, ultimately, labor and birth can unfold safely and as it needs to.

- I am surrounded and connected to love and support.
- I have a loving relationship with my partner and those around me.
- I create my reality, and my world is a loving, peaceful world.
- My body is beautiful.
- I experience abundance all around me.
- I am deeply attached to my baby.
- I love my baby.
- I feel gratitude for my pregnancy, my baby, and my family.
- I am safe and secure.
- I can openly and honestly communicate my intimate/sexual needs during pregnancy with my partner.

Write your own affirmations here:

- _____
- _____
- _____
- _____

*Affirmations for Your Partner:*
- I feel good about taking care of myself and my partner.
- I have everything I need to provide for and protect my family.
- I see strength in my partner.
- I am grateful for my partner and our relationship.
- I feel attached to my baby and my partner.
- I love our baby.
- I offer loving support to my partner freely and often.
- I express love freely.
- I experience abundance all around me.
- I create my reality, and my world is peaceful and joyful.
- I can openly and honestly communicate my intimate/sexual needs with my partner during her pregnancy.

Have your partner write his or her affirmations here:

- _____
- _____
- _____
- _____ ●

**ACTIVITY: FROM FEAR TO FAITH**

Write out a fear or worry that you have.

**I am worried about** _____

Next, rewrite this statement and turn it into an affirmation. For example, change "I fear that I will not be a good mother" to "I have all the resources and love I need to protect, nurture, and feel attached to my baby."

**My new affirmative statement:** _____

Now think of something that makes you feel content and grateful. Once you have connected to this feeling, repeat your new affirmation. Do this several times a day. ●

## More Resources for Developing a PMA

If you are finding it hard to develop a positive mental attitude for a better motherbaby bond, you are not alone. There are many helpful therapies with qualified practitioners that can help change the subconscious mind (your prewired brain). Here are just a few examples:

- **CBT (Cognitive Behavior Therapy):** This therapy produces excellent results at reprogramming the subconscious mind. CBT helps individuals take situations that may seem overwhelming and helps break them down into smaller parts so they become manageable. There is significant evidence that CBT improves attitude.

- **EMDR (Eye Movement Desensitization and Reprocessing):** This psychotherapy technique, which involves recalling past memories and tapping on energy points, might sound strange, but it has been widely researched and has proven to be a very effective way for people to deal with current or past trauma that may be affecting their lives. It helps to relieve psychological stress and can be used effectively when there appears to be significant barriers to internal happiness. For more information, visit *www.EMDRIA.org*.

- **Emotional Freedom Technique (EFT) and PSYCH-K:** These are both psychological techniques used to free the subconscious of mental and emotional barriers that prevent happiness. These techniques are based on mind-body medicine, as well as brain research, to help undo beliefs and traumas that are programmed into the subconscious mind. These therapies involve a technique similar to acupressure, which uses energy points, as well as applied kinesiology (muscle testing), to rewire the brain. To explore these therapies it is important to find qualified practitioners.

Your attachment pregnancy centers around creating a secure and safe bond between you and your baby. When you realize how deeply your attitude and emotions affect your developing baby and understand the nature of attachment, it becomes almost impossible not to "pay attention." You will find yourself more mindful and conscious of your thoughts, your attitude, and your baby. You can choose to proactively parent prenatally and create an attachment pregnancy with every thought you think.

# CHAPTER SUMMARY

Babies learn what they live, especially in the womb, and there is not a more crucial time for you to help your baby form a positive mental attitude and healthy perception of the world than during pregnancy. Your bond with your baby means that you are your child's first teacher. Having a positive mental attitude throughout pregnancy is the ultimate act of love for your child. Remember:

- Negative attitudes create stress in the body, and stress impacts every part of your pregnancy.

- Your thoughts dictate the development of your baby's brain in the womb, which will ultimately shape her perception of her world later in life.

- When you focus on developing a positive mental attitude during pregnancy, you create the most opportunity for an attachment pregnancy.

- Your body and mind are not separate, nor are your feelings separate from your baby's development. Having an attitude of gratitude creates the healthiest environment for pregnancy and your baby's development.

- You can teach your child to love life, embrace change, and look for the good, even in the unexpected, right from the start.

- Remember the three Rs to breaking the habit of negative thinking: Recognize it, Review it, and Replace it.

- Affirmations are positive statements of beliefs or truths that reflect your inner intentions and contribute to a positive mental attitude during pregnancy.

- If you're struggling to develop a PMA, look into CBT (Cognitive Behavior Therapy), EMDR (Eye Movement Desensitization and Reprocessing), EFT (Emotional Freedom Technique), and PSYCH-K. These therapies can strengthen your attachment pregnancy by changing your negative subconscious thoughts.

# CHAPTER 3

# Meditation During Pregnancy

> **"The present moment is filled with joy and happiness. If you are attentive, you will see it."**
> ~Thich Nhat Hanh, Zen Buddhist Monk

Whether you call it meditation, prayer, sitting quietly, quieting the mind, or being still, it all achieves the same result: stillness. Meditation allows you to tune deep within, connect to your baby, and become mindful of your internal world. Be-ing lays the foundation for successful meditation during an attachment pregnancy. Meditation or prayer allows you to develop insight to any questions you have, because you are in a mental state that allows you to be open to receiving answers. Meditation is like a two-way radio; as long as you are talking, you cannot hear any messages from the other side. You have to stop talking and become quiet to receive messages. These messages can come from within or from your source (your reason for being, God, etc.). The type of message you receive depends on your belief system and from where and how you seek guidance. You may or may not experience a gut reaction, a spiritual insight, or a mental thought. Either way, meditation clears your mind so that you become quiet enough to pay attention to your subconscious mind, your baby, and/or your source. From the quiet space of meditation, you can explore the thoughts and beliefs that will deepen the attachment to your baby. When you meditate you spend focused time with yourself and your baby. This one-on-one time helps you get to know your baby and promotes a sense of well-being and calmness that is integral to an attachment pregnancy.

## How Meditation Affects Attachment

If you want to do just one thing to benefit the health of your baby during your pregnancy, it should be to reduce stress as much as possible. Meditation is a simple, easily accessible way to eliminate stress, and it is available to you almost anywhere! Meditation helps the body and mind eliminate stress hormones, which is very important in pregnancy. When you are in a meditative state, you also release beneficial hormones (neurohormones and neurotransmitters) that your baby will receive through the placenta and later on through breastmilk. These little molecular messengers can help calm your baby, as well as help develop her emotional intelligence by sending her waves of love and other emotions. What could be better than a few moments a day when you send your baby all of the physical benefits of meditation, such as immune support, relaxation hormones, and emotional molecules of happiness? Isn't it exciting that you can have a positive impact on the future temperament of your child? But how exactly does this work? Let's take a closer look at the benefits of meditation.

### DHEA

Meditation can elevate DHEA, which is known as the "mother hormone" because it acts as a precursor to many other important hormones, including the male and female sex hormones. It is also an elemental hormone for pregnancy, for without DHEA, it's impossible for a baby to grow during pregnancy. It's known as a life-giving hormone. DHEA also increases the effectiveness of the immune system by increasing production of critical immune factors, such as T-cells, which are transferred to your baby during pregnancy.

## Melatonin

Meditation also stimulates the pineal gland, which secretes the hormone melatonin. Melatonin helps you sleep and helps your brain move into the deepest state of relaxation, known as the *alpha state*. When your brain is in an alpha state, your body can easily relax, repair itself, and increase its immune function. When you are well-rested and healthy, you have more energy to focus on bonding with your baby.

## Endorphins

Meditation also releases endorphins into the bloodstream. Endorphins are naturally produced opiates that help you feel good and reduce pain. During pregnancy, these endorphins are also sent to your baby. When you feel good, your baby feels good. Additionally, they help to positively influence your baby's brain and organ development.

## Psychological Benefits

Meditation also provides psychological benefits to both you and your baby. Research has associated meditation with creativity, empathy, concentration, and self-actualization. Your mind releases chemical messengers of emotions, called neuropeptides, or molecules of thought. These thought molecules communicate your emotional states to all of your organ systems so that you can best respond to any environment you are in. During pregnancy, these thought molecules pulse throughout the body, enter the placenta, and then are reproduced and delivered directly to your baby. Through these molecules of emotion you can communicate to your unborn baby. Your baby feels everything you feel and begins to develop his own emotional life based on your emotions. Though your baby is always receiving thought molecules from you, changing according to your emotional state, meditation is a time when you can focus on sending loving, positive, life-fulfilling thoughts to your baby. When your mind is calm and you focus your thoughts on love or another positive emotion, your baby is getting a large dose of positive molecules of thought. This is one of the ways that emotional intelligence—the way your baby begins to understand emotions and the world—is created in babies. By sending positive thought molecules during meditation, you can positively influence your baby's world and her future emotional health. Now that you know meditation is so beneficial for your attachment pregnancy, how do you do it? Read on . . .

## Pregnancy Meditation Guide

Meditation does not have to mean sitting in a yoga pose and chanting. It simply means having an opportunity to be in a space where you can quiet your mind, become still in your body, and connect to your source. Some people find that they can move into meditative states while walking in nature, running, or by simply sitting outside in their garden. There are many ways to become mindful of your internal world.

Meditation does not need to have many rules. Meditation and prayer are practiced around the world in many different traditions, in many different ways. There is no right or wrong way to do it. The key is that you practice in a manner that feels good to you. If you are a beginner to meditation and prayer, you might find it helpful to use a guided meditation. You will find one at the end of this chapter. Though there are countless practices, the following instructions can be used by any pregnant mother.

ACTIVITY: MEDITATION

This technique is simple, though initially it will involve conscious effort. With frequent practice, it will begin to become second nature.

- Sit where you can be warm and comfortable and have at least five to ten minutes to yourself. You don't have to sit cross-legged or even on the floor, but that is a commonly used meditation position. During pregnancy, as your belly gets larger, it may feel more comfortable if you place a folded towel or mat under your bottom. You can also lie down if you need to; just get comfortable. If meditating while lying down, you should lie on your left side to improve blood flow to your baby.

- Once you are comfortable, allow your spine to lengthen, and feel yourself sitting taller. If you are lying down, feel your body stretching out. If you wish, you can place one hand over your heart and one hand over your belly. This is a common pregnancy meditation posture, as it helps you visualize the connection between your heart and your baby.

- For a few minutes, simply focus on your breathing. Don't try to change it; just notice it. Allow thoughts to enter your mind, but instead of reacting to them, just let them go. It is very difficult to have a clear mind when you first begin to meditate. Becoming aware of your thoughts and simply observing them (instead of reacting emotionally to them) allows your mind to become calm.

- Tune in to what is happening with your baby. As you become still, notice if your baby begins to move or becomes still. Imagine looking inside and seeing your baby's face. Send love to your baby.

- Begin to slow your breath, pausing briefly between each inhale and exhale. As your breath slows, begin to become aware of your body, letting go of any tension you feel with each exhalation. Return your thoughts again to your baby, sending any loving messages you wish at this time. Allow yourself to feel gratitude for the bond between you and your baby. Feel the sensation of gratitude wash over you.

- You may also wish to consciously give an offering of gratitude to your body for supporting your baby during this pregnancy. Give thanks for your growing belly, which houses and protects your baby. Offer gratitude for your placenta, which nourishes your baby and sends your baby messages of love. Be grateful for your growing breasts, preparing to nurture and warm your baby. Honor all that your body is doing to create the motherbaby bond. Stay in this meditative space as long as you can. Once finished, notice how you feel. Take pleasure in knowing that you and your baby have benefited from this practice. Carry this feeling around with you all day. ●

## Guided Meditations

The following section includes a guided meditation that your partner or friend can read to you or that you can read to yourself. Guided meditations are scripts that can be used to help you get into a state of meditation and deep relaxation. It can be very helpful to use guided meditations when you are a beginner or when you are looking for a customized script for your meditation. For example, you can find guided meditations for relaxation in labor, for abundance, and even for increasing your milk supply when you breastfeed! It might be helpful to record yourself reading this meditation out loud so you can practice it anytime, including during your labor. If you choose to read to yourself, close your eyes and let your mind take you where it may after you have read the meditation. If you enjoy using guided meditations, there are many pregnancy and labor guided meditations you can find on the Internet.

## ACTIVITY: INTENTION-SETTING MEDITATION

This meditation is designed to help you listen to your inner voice, which is an essential tool for an attachment pregnancy. During meditation you can become aware of what your mind, body, spirit, and baby really need. When you become aware of these needs, you can set intentions—plans that help you move toward your higher purpose—to help you create change. This meditation is designed to be practiced while in a sitting position for comfort reasons.

- Allow your eyelids to close and your eyes to relax. Release any tension between your brows. Tune in to your breathing and to your baby. For the next few moments, simply allow yourself to listen to your breath. Don't try to change or manipulate your breathing. Simply notice your breathing. Become aware of how your breath flows through your body. Does your chest expand? Your belly? Is the inhalation or exhalation longer? Is there a pause between breaths, or does your breath loop into one continuous circle? Is there a place in your body where the breath seems to catch and pause, or does your breath flow evenly throughout your body? As you breathe, remember to tune in to your baby as well.
- Now that you have observed your breath, purposefully slow down your breathing. Intentionally inhale, bringing the breath into the body like delicious sips of air, filling a vessel. Fill the vessel of your body from lungs to diaphragm to abdomen. Allow for a short pause between inhalation and exhalation. Exhale slowly; feel the air pour out of your body, releasing, softening, letting go. Continue breathing in this manner for the next few breaths until you can let go of your thinking mind and simply allow the deep breath to move through the body without having to think about it.
- Begin to slowly bring your focus on the space between your brows, sometimes called the third eye. This space actually houses

the pineal gland, a fascinating gland that is stimulated in times of deep meditation. This gland releases hormones that help achieve a mental state of alpha, a relaxed state where your subconscious and conscious mind can meet. When this gland is stimulated, it cues your body into a deep sense of well-being and creativity.

- Bring your attention to this space between your brows. You may, in fact, wish to imagine that your breath is beginning to flow in and out through this space. As your breath moves through this space, it creates an opening for energy movement. Feel this space warming and energizing. Spend the next few moments simply focusing on this space and breathing in the manner that feels best to you.

- Now that you have stimulated your pineal gland, your body and mind are ready for intention setting. As you breathe deeply, invite an intention to present itself to you. Do not force an intention to come to you; simply invite it to manifest itself within your thoughts. Try not to judge the intention, and simply allow whatever your spirit needs to become present. It may seem odd or strange to you, but know that in this state of mindfulness, your subconscious mind is speaking to you.

- Once the intention is clear, feel your breath moving in and out through this thought. Invite the intention to manifest itself in your life. Imagine this intention becoming a part of your life, so that it becomes a part of you. Think about how this intention will enrich your pregnancy and the life of your baby. Feel gratitude for this intention being a part of your life.

- Return to your breath. Inhaling and exhaling, feeling relaxed and peaceful. As you allow your breath pattern to normalize, feel good about the intention you have set. Carry this feeling with you and your baby throughout the day. ●

Once you begin incorporating regular meditation into your life, you will find that it becomes an integral part of your day. Just like a daily practice of exercise or eating healthy foods, meditation is another way to take care of yourself and your baby. Additionally, it enhances the motherbaby bond, so get started today. As the Zen saying goes, you should sit in meditation for twenty minutes a day, unless you are busy—then you should sit for an hour.

# CHAPTER SUMMARY

Adopting a mindful approach to life allows you to strengthen the mother-baby bond, connect to your source, and become mindful of your internal world. Remember:

- Practicing meditation, prayer, and breathing awareness can help you move into a mindful state of Be-ing.

- There are many ways to become mindful of your internal world, including but not limited to meditation, walking in nature, running, and simply sitting outside in the garden.

- During meditation, your brain releases molecular messengers that can help calm your baby, as well as help develop her emotional intelligence by sending her waves of love and other emotions.

- Meditation during pregnancy increases beneficial hormones supportive to you and your baby.

- Meditation helps you communicate directly with your unborn baby.

# CHAPTER 4

# Conscious Agreement and Conscious Attachment

> "Before embarking on important undertakings, sit quietly, calm your senses and thoughts, and meditate deeply. You will then be guided by the great creative power of Spirit."
>
> ~Paramahansa Yogananda, Yogi and Guru

You make decisions every moment of every day. Whether these decisions are large or small, when you are pregnant every decision you make impacts your baby in some way. As we discussed in Chapter 1, the challenge during pregnancy is that you are often not in a space of mindfulness when making most of your decisions, which means that you are not practicing Be-ing, nor are you tuned in to your baby's needs. From the very moment of conception, you are your baby's advocate and protector. Learning how to be conscious of your decisions and their impact on your baby is a vital ingredient for the attachment pregnancy.

During your pregnancy, you will be asked to make many decisions regarding your healthcare. A term you may be exposed to in pregnancy books, your doctor's office, childbirth classes, or the hospital is *informed consent*. Informed consent is a legal term that means you are consenting to accept a medical procedure, and that you have been informed of all the benefits, risks, and alternatives to any treatment offered to you. This is meant to empower you as a patient; however, it fails to address the importance of conscious decision-making based on your own intuition, instincts, and gut feelings. Informed consent is made with the mind or intellect, but for a true attachment pregnancy you must go deeper, past your intellect, into Conscious Agreement, the act of making decisions based on deep inner listening and coming to an intuitive mind/body/spirit/baby agreement. Think about every decision you make as having potential consequences for your baby.

## Why Conscious Agreement?

Pregnancy is the ideal time to make decisions using Conscious Agreement, because it is all about making decisions that feel good at a gut level by choosing what is best for you and your baby in every moment. Conscious Agreement occurs when you are in collaboration with your inner wisdom, when every part of you says "Yes!" It's about moving into a space of trust and intuition. This can initially cause anxiety, because when you pay attention to your feelings and make decisions based on your inner wisdom, you are solely responsible for the decision and for the outcome. There is no one else to blame; you are the creator of everything that stems from that decision.

When you begin to develop the skill of being in Conscious Agreement for all of the decisions you make during pregnancy and beyond, your life will begin to move toward a different path; a path of less resistance and more opportunity, a place of deep trust and wisdom. You will be making decisions that support your attachment pregnancy and honor your bond to your baby. Doesn't this sound like a better path to follow?

How do you know when you are *not* acting in Conscious Agreement during pregnancy? Think of a time when you made an important decision and it did not feel quite right to you. You made a choice even when your inner voice disagreed. Did this decision really work out for you? You can also tell if you're not acting in Conscious Agreement when:

- You make a decision and something just feels wrong; your gut is telling you something is not right. Interesting note: your digestive system has neural tissue that responds to feelings and emotions. Paying attention to your "gut" reactions tells you what you think at an intuitive level.
- You experience uncomfortable physical symptoms, such as sleeplessness, stomachache, problems with concentration, or a general feeling of dis-ease.
- You feel detached from your baby.
- You continue to question your decision.

These physical signs are signals designed to alert you that your body, mind, spirit, and baby are not communicating in harmony. Your internal compass is telling you to go in one direction and yet you choose another path. You are functioning in a state of unconsciousness. If you feel this way, it is time to redirect and take the necessary steps to Conscious Agreement.

## Steps to Conscious Agreement

Conscious Agreement is a tool not only for your attachment pregnancy, but for your entire life. You can use this tool to help you make wise decisions as a mother, a patient (during labor and delivery), and even as a savvy consumer. During pregnancy, Conscious Agreement allows you to not only listen in to your own gut feelings, but also to pay attention to your baby's needs, through the motherbaby bond. Once your baby is born, you can begin teaching her this life tool to help her trust and follow her intuition as well. Conscious Agreement will help you make decisions based on your inner wisdom that you can always feel good about. There are four simple steps to practicing Conscious Agreement:

- Step One: Separate yourself from external influences.
- Step Two: Get quiet and pause.
- Step Three: Listen in.
- Step Four: Choose and commit!

To learn how to use these steps, read on.

### Step One: Separate yourself from external influences

This does not mean you have to go on retreat to the mountains or even leave the room. You can do this anywhere, anytime. For example, you can excuse yourself for a breath of fresh air, a bathroom break, or a glass of water and use this time to begin to redirect. You can also simply close your eyes. This separation is important, because people often make decisions based on the expectations of others and their own subconscious reactions to others.

Have you ever noticed how someone else's mood can actually influence your mood? Research shows that your brainwaves physically sync with the people around you. How does this happen? Well, your brain releases the same hormones as the people around you, which causes all of you to have similar thought patterns. In addition, your heartbeat syncs with those around you, which causes all of you to experience similar emotions. This syncing is called *entrainment*, a term you may have heard used by musicians. Why does the symphony all warm up together? Because when one musician finds the right note, this powerful musical resonance causes the other members of the orchestra to begin to synchronize their instruments, so everyone is playing in harmony. This is exactly what your brainwaves and heart rhythms do with the people around you. Remember the saying "misery loves company"? When you are around someone sad, you may begin to feel sad. The same is true for any other emotion, positive or negative.

When you remove yourself from others when you make a decision, you ensure that your decisions are made based on your own maternal intuition, not due to the influence of others. Be sure to separate yourself from external influences in order to stay tuned in to your internal "maternal" compass.

> **"Between stimulus and response there is a space. In that space is our power to choose our response. In our response lies our growth and our freedom."**
> ~Viktor Frankl, Holocaust Survivor, Neurologist,
> and Psychiatrist

### Step Two: Get quiet and pause

Take a moment, or a few, to quiet your mind, breathe deeply, and center your focus on the space around your heart, also known as your "heart space" or "sacred space." This step allows you to unplug from all external sources of influence and distraction and plug in to yourself and your own source. When you are in your heart space, your only influence is your source. Everything that emanates from this source is good, right, and in your—and your baby's—best interest.

It was recently discovered that the heart is as powerful as the brain, if not more so, when it comes to helping you choose the best course of action. In fact, research from the Institute of HeartMath has found that people make better decisions when they allow themselves to be tuned in to their heart space, which means that you should focus in on your heart space before you move on to the next step in achieving Conscious Agreement.

Why is the heart space so important? How does this work? The heart has a magnetic resonance approximately 5,000 times greater than that of the brain. This resonance is what allows your heart to sync with those around you. The heart also has neural tissue, or "thinking" tissue, that can read the environment around you. Your heart can perceive the emotional resonance of other people around you, to help you safely navigate your way through the world. During Conscious Agreement, it is important to leave the physical presence of other people, so that their emotions don't influence your decisions. The mere presence of others will cause your heart and emotions to begin to sync, which can change or influence your thinking.

**Step Three: Listen in**

When making a decision, think of all of the options in front of you. Imagine the possible outcomes of each option. Instead of making a snap decision, take the time to tune in and intentionally bring your baby into your thoughts. How do you feel, both physically and emotionally, when you think about your options? Which option feels right? Which option brings *you*—not other people—the most peace? Also, take this time to honor the motherbaby bond. After all, your decisions deeply affect your baby and her long-term health and happiness. As you visualize your options, place a hand over your belly and consciously consider your baby. Does this feel right for both of you? Keep in mind that the option that feels right for you and your baby may not be the easiest route; in fact, it may be a difficult path. But if you look back at your past decisions, you will likely find that some of your more challenging decisions led to the most personal growth.

**Step Four: Choose and commit!**

Now it's time to make the decision that feels right, and commit yourself to that decision. You are in control. You make your own decisions. You are responsible. Let go of feeling a sense of guilt for other people's reactions. You are only responsible for your own feelings. Just as you have the opportunity to shift your attitude and choose your emotional response to situations, so do all of the other people in your life. You are not responsible for the feelings of others. At every moment, you have the opportunity to choose Conscious Agreement for yourself—and your baby. By consciously choosing to live in the moment, and not in the bondage of your subconscious mind, you choose a lifetime bond with your baby through an attachment pregnancy.

## Medical Tests in Pregnancy and Conscious Agreement

When using Conscious Agreement for decisions about prenatal testing and medical decisions for you and your baby, remember that the goal is to be in Conscious Agreement with yourself *and* your baby. Over the course of your pregnancy, you will likely be asked to have a variety of tests ranging from blood work (monitoring pregnancy health) to amniocentesis (monitoring health of baby) to ultrasound (monitoring baby's organs, developmental markers, placental health, etc.). Each test can give you information about your pregnancy, your baby, and her health, but some tests carry a certain level of risk. Prior to your prenatal visits, you can use Conscious Agreement to help you make decisions about which tests are right for you and your baby. Here are some general questions to ask yourself to help you decide what decisions feel right:

- Is there a benefit to my baby? To myself? To my pregnancy, labor, and birth?
- Is there a risk to my baby? To myself? To my pregnancy, labor, and birth?
- How does having this test make me feel?
- Are the results of this particular test very accurate, or does it have a high false-positive rate?

- Will the knowledge about the results potentially change my bond with my baby? Do I want it to? Can it help me/my baby in any way?
- Will the knowledge this test provides alter the outcome of my attachment pregnancy? Would I change anything about my care, care provider, place of birth, or birth plan depending on the results?
- Can the diagnosis/disease this test screens for be treated effectively during/after pregnancy?
- Do I feel pressured to have the test? Is that impacting my decision?
- Are there any alternatives to the test?
- Am I in a high-risk category? Does that change my decision to have the test?
- Am I making my decision from a place of fear or a place of trust?
- What am I specifically afraid of? How might I handle the situation if my fears were realized?
- Would I feel better knowing the results?
- Is not knowing whether my child has the specific condition to be tested for affecting my ability to bond with my baby?

When you begin to make decisions in Conscious Agreement, you will change the outcome of your pregnancy. Throughout pregnancy and parenting you will be faced with daily choices. Making these choices in Conscious Agreement ensures that you are giving your baby the best that you have to give.

## Conscious Attachment

While making decisions in Conscious Agreement during pregnancy can help ensure that you are doing what is right for you and your baby throughout pregnancy and beyond, you also want to make certain that you are consciously and directly communicating and connecting to your baby as often as you can. This is called *Conscious*

*Attachment* and is another important practice along the journey to an attachment pregnancy. Your baby is becoming a conscious being from the early moments of conception. She has neural connections in her brain and begins to feel all that you are feeling as she grows. Your consciousness of your world changes the very development of her brain and all of her organs, which means that the more often you practice Conscious Attachment, the more often your baby is experiencing the deepest loving attachment to you that is possible.

## The Steps to Conscious Attachment

Conscious Attachment allows you to consciously connect with and bond to your baby, anytime and anywhere, and ensures that you stay connected to what is most important during pregnancy: the motherbaby bond. The steps to Conscious Attachment are simple and easy to practice. They include:

- Step One: Get quiet and pause
- Step Two: Get in touch
- Step Three: Communicate
- Step Four: Promise

To learn more, read on.

### Step One: Get quiet and pause

Throughout the day, it is easy to become distracted and forget about the attachment to your baby. Life is often busy and hectic, and that means being conscious becomes more difficult. To truly have an attachment pregnancy, you must consciously attach to your baby. The moment you become aware of your disconnect is a moment of awakening for you and your baby. Take hold of this moment, become quiet, and pause. Remember who you really are at your core and become aware of your heart space.

### Step Two: Get in touch

Place one hand over your heart and one hand over your belly. Slow your breath and become aware of the beating of your heart and the presence of your baby. It is common for mothers to rub their bellies when they tune in to their baby, and you may find yourself doing this as well. This is called *effleurage*. In fact, seeing other mothers practicing effleurage can remind you to move into Conscious Attachment.

### Step Three: Communicate

Direct loving attention and intentions toward your baby. Remember that you are sharing molecules of emotions with your baby, and everything you feel, your baby feels. Send your baby any loving messages you wish during this time. It is an opportunity to bond and openly communicate with your baby. Accept and experience your baby's love for you.

### Step Four: Promise

As you experience this intimate connection to your baby, realize how important taking this time to bond with your baby is to your attachment pregnancy. Make a promise to yourself and your baby to stay in this space as long and as often as you can.

Incorporating Conscious Agreement and Conscious Attachment into your life will allow you to use and more importantly trust your amazing maternal instincts to protect and nurture your baby. These practices allow you to strengthen your relationship with your baby and will help her trust the world she will be born into. There is nothing more sacred and beautiful than the bond between mother and child, and by practicing Conscious Agreement and Conscious Attachment, you are loving yourself and your baby and consciously embracing an attachment pregnancy.

# CHAPTER SUMMARY

Consciousness during pregnancy is the act of choosing to practice Conscious Agreement and Conscious Attachment to your baby, where you make mindful decisions based on deep inner listening and come into an intuitive mind/body/spirit agreement.

- The decisions you and your partner make during pregnancy either strengthen or weaken the attachment to your baby.

- Conscious Agreement is about choosing what is best for you and your baby in every moment by using your inner wisdom.

- Your body will give you physical signals, such as a stomachache, when you are not acting in Conscious Agreement.

- The steps to Conscious Agreement are: Step One: Separate yourself from external influences. Step Two: Get quiet and pause. Step Three: Listen in. Step Four: Choose and commit.

- Remember that people in your life can influence your decisions because your heart syncs with those around you.

- When making decisions about medical tests and healthcare for you and your baby during pregnancy, remember to practice Conscious Agreement for the best outcome.

- The more often you are practicing Conscious Attachment, the more often your baby is experiencing the deepest loving attachment to you that is possible.

- The steps to Conscious Attachment are: Step One: Get quiet and pause. Step Two: Get in touch. Step Three: Communicate. Step Four: Promise.

Chapter 4: Conscious Agreement and Conscious Attachment **61**

# CHAPTER FIVE

# Building Supportive Relationships

"Every issue, belief, attitude, or assumption is precisely the issue that stands between you and your relationship to other human beings and between you and yourself."

~Gita Bellin, Performance Consultant, Facilitator, Mentor, and Coach

You and your baby are not in a vacuum during pregnancy; instead, you both are affected by every person with whom you have a relationship. Your relationships, including your relationship to self, and the emotions that you experience as a result of those relationships, change the lives of both you and your baby during pregnancy. When someone you are involved with makes you happy, your baby experiences happiness. Likewise, when you have an angry or frustrating encounter with someone, your baby feels these emotions as well. Your emotional health changes the development of your baby's brain and shapes your baby's personality. When you become aware of how people make you and your baby feel, you have the opportunity to consciously choose who you spend time with during your attachment pregnancy. When you extend gratitude for these supportive relationships, you open the door for even greater good during your pregnancy.

## Relationship to Self

The word *relationship* likely brings to mind those people outside of yourself—your partner or other people in your life. However, the most important relationship that you will ever have during attachment pregnancy is the relationship you have with yourself. This is a relationship that begins with self-awareness. You must first love and understand yourself before you can truly experience the motherbaby bond and, in fact, there is never a more critical period to love and understand yourself than when you choose to become a parent. Your self-love for and relationship with yourself is the very foundation for your child's emotional development. It is true that children learn what they live, and you are your child's first teacher.

### Listen to Your Thoughts

How often do you really listen to your thoughts? This is the beginning of true self-awareness. Listening to your thoughts with an open mind and without judgment allows you to truly become aware of your belief systems. As you grow in self-awareness, you will better understand the foundation of many of your beliefs, perceptions, and habits. It will allow you to get to know yourself. Examining your thoughts and belief systems gives you an opportunity to look deep inside and think about changing the things that no longer make sense as you become a mother. Knowing yourself, who you are, what you want, and why you want it, gives you an opportunity to move into Conscious Agreement with yourself and your world.

Simply put, no one knows *you* better than *you*. You already have the answers; there is no need to seek external input.

## Explore Your Beliefs

Your beliefs shape every relationship that you have—including the one that you have with yourself and your baby. A deep look at your beliefs, where they came from, and if they are serving you or hurting you is another step toward healthy self-awareness. Remember, a belief is when your mind accepts something whether it is true or not, and your beliefs are generated from the memories of your past. These are the stories you tell yourself to make sense of the world. These are also the stories that will shape your baby.

### What Is Your Story?

Are you the conscious author of your own story, or did other people and the events and other things that happened to you write your story a long time ago? Your family of origin and the memories you hold about your past may have a great impact on your thoughts, feelings, and beliefs about yourself. It's important not to underestimate the extent that these beliefs impact your sexuality, pregnancy, birth, and parenting behaviors, because these belief systems have the potential to in fact change your baby's health outcomes, personality, and belief systems. Your core beliefs, like it or not, attract the people, events, and situations in your life.

If you have an attitude of fear or shame around pregnancy/ birth/parenting, this can manifest into fearful and shameful experiences. Many children grow up in families where sexuality and all things related to reproduction (menstruation, pregnancy, etc.) have an element of shame or embarrassment associated with them. This negative perception of your body and the process of womanhood can and does affect the way you conceive, grow, birth, and parent your babies. Often women are unconscious about what they really believe concerning their bodies and pregnancy because these beliefs are held in the subconscious mind. Now, during your attachment pregnancy, is the perfect time to begin to change the way you've been subconsciously thinking about things and to tell your story as you wish it to be. Create your life with the intentions you desire for yourself and your baby.

Recognize that it can be common to move into a state of mind of victimization, where you blame others for your thoughts when you uncover belief systems that don't feel good. But allowing yourself to stay in a state of victimization or self-pity actually wires these beliefs deeper into your subconscious. It is critical to be committed to change, and to give yourself an opportunity to move into a state of gratitude or appreciation every time you feel challenged by these beliefs. Notice your feelings (observe them), honor them (do not react to them), and then move into a state of gratitude as often as you can (gratitude is discussed in more detail later in this chapter). This is being mindful. As you move forward, keep in mind that it is difficult to do this work, but the more you practice changing your fears/unwanted beliefs into opportunities, the easier it will become. After all, uncovering your belief systems presents an opportunity for you and for your baby. When you break the cycle of unwanted beliefs, you change the world and the future for your child and future generations.

> "We build our lives on the foundation of our stories. The more we invest in a story, the more important it becomes to continue investing in that story, even after it is clear the story no longer works."
>
> ~Bruce Lipton, Biologist and Author of
> *Spontaneous Evolution: Our Positive Future*

Answer the questions and follow the steps in the following activity to begin to edit your current beliefs if they don't tell the story of the life you want to live and the parent you want to be.

## ACTIVITY: EXPLORE YOUR BELIEFS

Here is a list of questions to help you explore your innermost beliefs so you can choose to change those beliefs that do not support an attachment pregnancy. In the exploration of your belief systems and its origins, it is crucial that you recognize the importance of changing the beliefs that do not reflect what you *want*. This exercise is designed to help you:

- Become more conscious of your belief systems and how they were created
- Determine whether your current beliefs will benefit you and your baby
- Create positive change at a deep level

Follow each of the steps in this activity to move forward.

### Step One

Sit in a quiet space alone and allow yourself to journal freely the answers to the following questions. Try not to over-think your answers or mentally edit them; just allow yourself to write freely as the thoughts come to you. Some of the memories you uncover may be painful or uncomfortable. This is exactly why you want to recognize them and then move into a space of change. After this exercise, if you feel that you need help processing and changing these beliefs, please review the therapies mentioned in Chapter 2. In particular, the techniques of EFT and PSYCH-K are specifically designed to change belief systems at a subconscious level relatively quickly. The questions you need to answer to begin to change your story are:

- What things did your family and friends say to you about your body when you were a child? Were adolescence, sexuality, and body changes openly and positively discussed? What feelings do you remember having about your changing body as you grew up?
- What did the women in your family share with you or keep from you about their births and their bodies? How did that make you feel?
- What did your father or other men/boys in your life say about your body? Pregnancy? Childbirth? Sex? How did that make you feel?
- What was the overall attitude toward adolescence, sexuality, pregnancy, and parenting where you grew up? Do you feel it was positive or negative?
- Why do you want to have a child? Why do you want to be a parent? What are your fears about having a child?
- What can you give to your child? What do you want to give to your child?
- How were babies/children seen in your family? Is this something you want to embrace in your own family? Why or why not?
- How do your parents and siblings feel about you having a child? How do your closest friends feel about your pregnancy?
- How does your partner feel about having a child? Have you actually discussed his or her feelings, or are you assuming what those feelings are?

## Step Two

Now that you have answered these questions, reread your answers. Do your answers reflect who you want to be in this pregnancy and as a mother? Which answers are supportive of an attachment pregnancy? Mark the answers that reflect the ideals that you want to pass on to your child.

## Step Three

Make a list of all the beliefs you wish to change and why you want to change them.

### Step Four

Rewrite the beliefs you wish to change into positive affirmations. Repeat these affirmations to yourself daily. You can also print them out and post them around your house. The daily practice of using affirmations will help shift your subconscious mind. See Chapter 2 for more on affirmations. ●

## Relationship to Others

Relationships are what the human connection is all about. Your family, your friends and community, your coworkers, your spiritual fellowship, and even your healthcare team all affect how you think, how you feel, and what you do during your pregnancy. Your relationships have a direct impact on your attachment to your baby, as they can influence how you are feeling and acting. In fact, one of the first critical mothering tasks you have is determining your boundaries between you and your baby and the people in your life. Having an attachment pregnancy means surrounding yourself with loving, supportive relationships, and this is the time mothers commonly become conscious of their relationships with others, their relationship with their source, and their relationships with their healthcare providers.

### Look at Your Relationships

To have a strong attachment pregnancy, you need to ask yourself:

- Who in your life provides you with the support, love, and connection that will ultimately lead to a healthy pregnancy and a happy baby?
- Which relationships in your life should you re-examine?

Who you allow in your life is very important. You and your baby are affected and influenced by the people that surround you. There is no better time than now to start to look at which relationships enrich your life and which relationships keep you from being the best mother you can be. The attitudes of the people around you are contagious, and the people who surround you during pregnancy directly affect the health and happiness of the child you will raise. Having conscious relationships is crucial to a happy and fulfilled pregnancy and life. Your relationships change the experience of your pregnancy and impact your ability to bond with your baby. You have the power and responsibility to consciously choose your relationships. It may be impossible to eliminate all unsupportive people in your life, but it is possible to establish firm boundaries.

## Set Personal Boundaries

What are personal boundaries? Personal boundaries are a set of limitations that you have for your physical and emotional health that you expect others to be respectful of, and they are healthy and necessary for an attachment pregnancy. When you have healthy personal boundaries, you are able to teach your children to have healthy personal boundaries. Creating healthy boundaries means taking an honest look at your relationships. When you don't know who you are or what you want, it is impossible to have healthy boundaries. Does it feel like your relationships are in Conscious Agreement with who you are, or who you want to be? Does it feel like your relationships are supportive of an attachment pregnancy? As you figure out what relationships are strong and supportive, keep in mind:

- It's okay to say "no."
- Tell yourself that *you* and your baby matter the most.

- You are not responsible for other people's feelings.
- Others are not responsible for *your* feelings either, nor should they have to feel the same way about situations that you do.
- Loving someone does not mean you have to engage in a relationship with them.

It is normal and expected that certain people in your life may be resistant to the healthy boundaries that you set up around your relationships. This can be challenging. However, you will find that the more you set boundaries and create healthier relationships, the happier you (and your baby) will be. You will also find that setting these boundaries will enable you to have more emotional energy to direct to your attachment pregnancy.

## The Sacred Circle of Support

Imagine yourself and your baby surrounded by the people in your life. Take a look around at all of these individuals and select those who are the most supportive and loving in their interactions with you during this pregnancy. This is your sacred circle of support, or your inner circle. This inner circle is a sacred space where you are in control. You decide who is in your inner circle. Why do you need to define this group of people? You need to know who plays what role in your life when you begin to identify your personal boundaries with everyone in your life. Those in your inner circle should make you feel safe and supported.

This inner circle might include your partner, your close family and friends, and those who are on your spiritual support team. As you reflect on your inner circle, notice that these are the individuals you should be closest to during pregnancy. These special individuals are there of your choosing, not just because of their relationship to you or because they are your neighbors or coworkers. They are in this sacred circle because they lift you up, enrich your pregnancy, and encourage your bond with your baby.

Now that you have chosen your inner circle, look at the people in your life who are left. These individuals comprise varying levels of outer circles, based on how close you want to be to them. These circles contain people you may wish to have more distance from at times. These people may drain you emotionally, may cause you stress, or you may simply not feel as close to them as those in your inner circle. Additionally, while you may have a deep emotional connection with some people in your outer circle, that connection may not be supportive for you. Defining your sacred circle of support, and identifying those in the inner and outer circles, is one way you can determine who you need to set firm boundaries with and maintain distance from during your attachment pregnancy. Note: Just because someone is not in your inner circle does not mean you don't love them. Your inner circle should simply be made up of those who give positive energy to you and your baby instead of taking energy away from you. It is important to recognize whether an individual is in your inner or outer circle when calling on that person for support.

Throughout your life your circle of support will change. You change as you grow, therefore your needs change as well as your relationships. Those in your inner circle when you were younger can be completely different from those in your inner circle now. Expect your inner circle to change again significantly after the birth of your baby. This can be troubling as you begin to realize that your inner circle has changed because you are changing. Out of habit, you may call on people for support who should have migrated to your outer circles. Pay attention, and take time to redefine your circles of support as needed.

## Gratitude in Relationships

When you are in a state of gratitude, your heart is open. It is in this state of gratitude that you are able to give and receive love and feel the closest to your baby. The act of gratitude is magnetic. Think of yourself and others as a magnet; you always draw to yourself what you are feeling/expressing. When you are grateful for the relationships you have with yourself and others, other people experience that appreciation and love. They are then likely to reciprocate love and appreciation. This reciprocity strengthens the relationships you have and improves your emotional state during your attachment pregnancy.

Resistance is the opposite of gratitude. It means that you are placing your focus on what you don't want in your life versus what you do want in your life. You get what you give. If you are focusing on behaviors and events in your relationships that you don't want, you actually draw those situations to yourself and your baby. Gratitude can be thought of as acceptance. When you are in a state of gratitude (acceptance versus resistance), you are in the optimal state to give and receive love. This is the best state in which to experience an attachment pregnancy and also the optimal state to attract the relationships that will benefit you and your baby.

Consider these scenarios of acceptance and resistance:

**Scenario one:** I can no longer eat fast food and drink soda as often as I like. I know making these choices will help nourish and nurture my growing baby. I love how my pregnancy has caused me to make overall better choices for my nutrition. I embrace this opportunity to love myself and my baby by making the best nutrition choices. (Acceptance)

**Scenario two:** All I want to do is eat a double cheeseburger with fries and a soda. I feel so deprived and irritated that I can't eat what I want to. I can't wait until this pregnancy is over. (Resistance)

Which of these scenarios opens the door to goodness in your life and is supportive of your attachment pregnancy?

When you are in a state of gratitude, it heightens your perceptions. It opens your eyes to the goodness of life all around you. It changes the way you see people, events, and situations in your world. When you are grateful, you open yourself up to more good, and by opening up to good, you attract it. Isn't this the world you wish your baby to be born into—a world of gratitude?

"We can only be said to be alive in those moments when our hearts are conscious of our treasures."

~Thornton Wilder, Pulitzer Prize–Winning Novelist

# CHAPTER SUMMARY

Your relationships—both with yourself and with others—are a reflection of your inner world and influence your reality and the health and development of your baby. Developing healthy personal boundaries and practicing gratitude in all of your relationships is a strong foundation for an attachment pregnancy. Remember:

- Your self-love and relationship to yourself is the very foundation for your child's emotional development.

- Examining your thoughts and belief systems gives you an opportunity to look deep inside and think about changing the things that no longer make sense as you become a mother.

- Edit your current beliefs if they don't tell the story of the life you want to live and the parent you want to be. Your belief systems have the potential to change your baby's health outcomes, personality, and belief systems.

- Having an attachment pregnancy means surrounding yourself with loving, supportive relationships. There is no better time than now to start to look at which relationships enrich your life and which relationships keep you from being the best mother you can be.

- When you have healthy personal boundaries, you are able to teach your child or children to have healthy personal boundaries.

- The individuals in your sacred circle of support should be there of your choosing and make you feel safe and supported. Pay attention, and give yourself permission to redefine your circles of support as needed.

- When using gratitude as a basis for all of your relationships, you are most able to give and receive love and feel closest to your baby.

# PART 2

# Observing: The First Trimester of Pregnancy

## B **O** N D

### O stands for Observing

"Listen to what you know
instead of what you fear."

~RICHARD BACH, Author of *Jonathan Livingston Seagull*

The first trimester is often an exciting and overwhelming time for most mothers. You may find yourself ecstatic about growing your family one moment, and then exhausted from all that there is to do. You will likely also begin to become more keenly aware of everything that is happening around you. This process of becoming more mindful and aware is about observing your life from the perspective of a mother. These observations and how you react to everything in your world is a pivotal part of an attachment pregnancy.

In this part, you'll learn how to change your mind so that you are observing your environment instead of reacting to your environment. Observing and changing is a building block for an attachment pregnancy and, in fact, research shows that a mother's brain is actually changing, creating new connections that allow her to "sense" her environment in new ways. For example, your sense of smell is heightening to help you observe your environment to keep your baby safe from things that could be toxic or harmful. As you begin to become more mindful of your world and create Conscious Agreement with everything in your life, your baby receives all of the benefits. You will begin to place your focus and your attention on those things that please you, that you are grateful for, and that make you feel fully alive and loved. When you consciously align with mindfulness, you have the opportunity for a deeper bond with your baby, because you are actually using a part of your brain that makes you feel and act more maternal. How can you use the skill of observing in your attachment pregnancy? Find out in the following chapters.

# CHAPTER 6

# What Is Observing?

> "To acquire knowledge, one must study; but to acquire wisdom, one must observe."
> ~Marilyn vos Savant, National Columnist and Author

How you observe the world will influence your attachment pregnancy and your baby's health. In fact, recent studies show that the more mindful and observant a mother becomes during her pregnancy, the less likely she is to experience prenatal depression. Pregnant mothers practicing mindfulness are also more likely to be able to manage stress effectively and have a higher degree of attachment to their babies. While it might be normal to feel guilty about some unconscious decisions you might have previously made, it is time to let guilt go. It is time to create change through observing.

## Why During Pregnancy?

Pregnancy is a time to begin to become aware of everything in your environment in order to deepen your attachment to your baby. As the bond to your baby grows you become more observant, knowing that everything that goes on in your world impacts your baby. The hormonal shift that takes place during pregnancy causes a magnification of your maternal protection instincts. This causes you to be hyperaware of how everyone in your life makes you feel, and in turn makes your baby feel. The changes in your body make you more aware of your baby and the importance of everything you do during pregnancy. You begin to pay more attention to what you eat and how often you exercise. Additionally, the importance of your spiritual life or relationship to your source also can become increasingly significant. The attachment pregnancy results in you becoming the observer of everything in your life, which only helps to deepen your bond to your baby.

Your ability to become more mindful as the observer of your environment allows you to consciously make better choices for your pregnancy. Before you can change an action or relationship that is unhealthy for you and your baby, you first have to observe that it is happening and recognize your desire for change. For example, many pregnant women will drive themselves to exhaustion during pregnancy to complete everything on their "to-do" list. They will continue this behavior in spite of the health consequences and increased stress levels. When mothers become conscious and observe the toll that this type of behavior is actually taking on them, the motherbaby bond, and their relationships, they are more likely to make better choices, such as napping, delegating responsibility, and letting go.

Keep in mind that during pregnancy, your world-view is being sent as molecular messages to your baby. This affects your baby's development and your baby's emotional health, or EQ (emotional quotient). Your body is a direct reflection of how your mind observes the world and, if you constantly perceive your world as a threat, your body reacts with stress hormones and creates dis-ease. This means your baby is also experiencing stress when you are. If you see the world as harmonious, your body is also in a state of harmony, as is your baby. You have tremendous power and opportunity during your pregnancy to change your life and the life of your baby. When gratitude, peace, and joy are rooted in your state of being, your baby will grow in a state of optimal health. Remember, these states of mind allow for a deeper connection with your baby, as you are more tuned in to a maternal state of mind.

## What's Up, Baby?

Your baby becomes who you *are* during pregnancy. Observing all aspects of who you are and who you want to become are the foundational keys to attachment pregnancy during the first trimester. Observing encompasses everything that you observe in the world and how you think and feel about your environment—about stress, routine medical tests in pregnancy, common physical discomforts, the food you eat, and the people and support systems around you. Most importantly, your observation of your baby over the first trimester is the critical component of attachment pregnancy. So let's take a look at what your baby is doing over the next twelve weeks and how her development can help with your motherbaby bond. Please note that your baby's developmental milestones will happen based on your family genetics and your environment. Therefore, the milestones can occur at slightly different times. This is why the weeks seem to overlap in the developmental periods below.

### Weeks One to Three:

During this time period, your baby develops into an embryo and implants herself into the endometrial lining of your uterus. The first nerve cells begin to develop. The heart forms long before the brain does. This is due to the fact that the heart is actually the regulatory organ of the body's sensory development. The heart has neural tissue, which helps your baby react and perceive her environment and begin to create her bond to you.

## Weeks Three to Ten:

During weeks three through ten, the placenta, the physical connection between you and your baby, has fully formed. Your baby has begun to develop all of her essential organs. Her brain has divided into five vesicles, and 100,000 nerve cells are developing every minute. Her heart starts beating. Her nipples, toes, and external genitals begin to form. Your baby's first sensitivity to touch begins. By the end of this period, your baby is moving all around, swallowing, and making hand-to-mouth movements.

## Weeks Ten to Twelve:

Your baby measures approximately 1 to 3 inches. Her face and ears have fully formed features and her limbs lengthen. Her eyelids are formed and closed. She can make a fist. She is sensitive to touch. She responds to your laughter, coughing, and loud sounds. Your baby also begins to determine her sense of balance and her sense of where she is in the world. At this stage, your baby is becoming more emotionally aware of her connection to you. When you start to think about how your baby is developing as a person, you become more tuned in and attached to her. She becomes real in a very physical and emotional way.

During the first trimester, as your baby grows and your capacity to mother develops, the gift of keen observation has been placed in your hands. Take the opportunity to pay attention as often as you can to enhance your bond with your baby. When you choose the gift of conscious observation, you choose the path of the attachment pregnancy.

# CHAPTER SUMMARY

The way that you observe your world and respond in kind will influence your ability to feel deeply attached to your baby. The more present and observant you are during pregnancy, the more you are aware of what you and your baby really need. Remember:

- The hormonal shift of pregnancy causes you to be hyperaware of how everyone and everything in your life makes you feel, and in turn makes your baby feel. These changes make you more aware of your baby and the importance of everything you do during pregnancy.

- Before you can change an action or relationship that is unhealthy for you and your baby, you first have to observe that it is happening and recognize your desire for change.

- When you consciously align with mindfulness, you have the opportunity for a deeper bond with your baby, because you are actually using a part of your brain that makes you feel and act more maternal.

- During pregnancy, your world-view is being sent as molecular messages to your baby. You choose whether your body and your baby are residing in stress or harmony.

- When you start to think about how your baby is developing as a person, you become more tuned in and attached to her.

# CHAPTER 7

# Stress Reduction During Pregnancy

> **"In the end, these things matter most: how well did you love, how fully did you live, how deeply did you learn to let go?"**
> ~Siddhartha Gautama, the Buddha

Stress is simply your body's reaction to unique events in your life. Not all stress is negative. In fact, there is eustress (positive stress) as well as distress (negative stress). Both forms of stress are designed to help your body safely travel through the world. When you experience something that demands attention, your body begins to prepare for this new experience. Your brain releases the stress hormones adrenaline and cortisol, which prepare your body for action. Your body reroutes circulation from its core to your extremities and muscle groups, your heart rate increases, your focus becomes narrow, your blood pressure rises, your digestion slows, and you get a spike of energy. This is often called "fight or flight."

In recent years, for the pregnant woman, this state has been called "tend or befriend," because instead of a mother wanting to engage in a fight or run away, she becomes very task-oriented, increases caretaking activity, and uses her social skills to negotiate relationships to protect herself and her baby at any cost. These types of activities ensure that mother and baby are in a safe place and well cared for. This response is due to your mothering instincts and proof of the attachment that has formed between you and your baby. You should avoid staying consistently in a "tend or befriend" state, which means you need to reduce and/or manage your stress as much as possible. How can you observe your stress and use this observation to reduce your stress levels during pregnancy? How does stress really affect you and your pregnancy anyway? Let's find out.

## Is Stress Dangerous?

You may be surprised to learn that acute or short-term stress during pregnancy is not harmful for your body, or even your baby. In fact short bursts of stress, which quickly and completely resolve and return your body to a state of normalcy, actually prepare your baby for stress resiliency throughout her life.

What can be damaging to your and your baby's health is when acute stress turns into chronic stress. This is when your body begins reacting to most things in your environment in a distress mode. For example, when in the state of "tend or befriend," your focus is often on taking care of others instead of caring for yourself. Examples include being frequently in a frenzied state of housekeeping, errand running, and tending to chores. When too much attention is placed on these activities, it can be a sign of distress. During chronic stress, your body continuously releases the stress hormone cortisol, which is not healthy for your pregnancy or your baby. Some studies even show that increased anxiety and stress can decrease the feeling of attachment between mother and baby. Your body can either make DHEA, the crucial pregnancy hormone, or it can make cortisol, the stress hormone. DHEA is the main hormone that maintains and supports a healthy pregnancy. When your body is busy making cortisol, DHEA production is compromised. Chronic release of cortisol also increases your risk of prenatal depression, decreases generation of new cells, reduces memory, and reduces the ability to learn new things (an important skill during parenting).

## Perceived Stress

Perceived stress also impacts your and your baby's genes. Your genes have telomeres, areas of protection on the end of the DNA strand, which protect the gene's chromosomes from deterioration. When you are exposed to high levels of stress, or chronic stress, these telomeres are damaged. While your baby is developing, ideally she is in a low and managed stress environment, so that her chromosomes can grow healthy and strong. Interestingly, new research is showing that the enzyme that protects telomeres (telomerase) can be increased by feelings of compassion and acts of care toward others.

## Pregnancy and Stress

The good news is that, as a natural response to pregnancy, many pregnant women have a reduced stress reaction to stressful events. Your body is designed to protect and bond with your baby, so there are natural mechanisms on board to protect you both. During pregnancy, your body begins to respond to normal daily stressors in an entirely different way. Your brain actually changes, as do the levels of hormones it produces. Mothers are designed to become calmer, gentler, more loving, and nurturing as a result of pregnancy. One of the ways your body does this is by enabling your brain to deal with stress better.

However, while your body is likely providing some protection against stress, it is still your job to observe your environment and reduce potential stressful situations as much as you can. Pregnancy is a perfect time to be compassionate toward yourself, your baby, your family, and your community, as your pregnancy hormones, such as oxytocin and estrogen, increase loving feelings. Hugging someone, laughing, deeply listening to someone you care about, cooking and sharing a meal: all these things will benefit you and your baby! It's so simple, really.

## Benefits of Stress Reduction

You have the power to improve your life and your baby's life by committing yourself to stress reduction. Rather than becoming more anxious about stress, you can choose to think, *I have the power to reduce the risk of all of these things by taking care of myself. I can quiet my mind. I can take a few moments to do deep breathing. I can take a walk, do yoga, smile, and yawn* (a significant stress-reducer). *I have all the power. I can change my mind!* The activities just mentioned can change the outcome of your pregnancy and increase attachment. Best of all, they are simple and accessible. Focus on the opportunity you have during pregnancy to make change instead of the risks of being chronically stressed. Here are just a few ways lowering your stress can benefit you and your baby:

- Increased sense of connection between you and your baby
- Reduced risk of preterm birth
- Reduced risk of baby born small for gestational age
- Reduced risk of depression in the mother
- Development of a mature hippocampus in your baby (the emotional hub of the brain, which regulates hormones)
- Normal physical development in early infancy
- Increased cognitive scores for your infant
- Normal stress threshold for your baby (babies become stressed less often)

- Reduced risk of your baby's brain becoming habituated to stress hormones like ACTH and cortisol, which make her feel unsafe and scared
- Higher IQ
- Decreased behavioral problems in childhood and adolescence
- Reduced risk of your baby developing certain diseases (such as heart disease, obesity, diabetes) and neurodevelopmental disorders (such as autism, bipolar disease, and schizophrenia) later in life

With all of the benefits of having a low-stress pregnancy, why not take action and work to reduce your stress levels?

## How to Reduce Stress

Reducing stress does not have to be stressful. There are very simple and easy ways to manage your stress levels. There is no way to eliminate all stress from your life, but you can manage it. Things that are proven to reduce stress are: optimism, supportive relationships, meditation, yoga, smiling, yawning, and deep-breathing techniques. In this section, you will find some techniques and activities that you can use anywhere and anytime during your attachment pregnancy.

### Use the Four As

You also can use the four As of stress reduction—Avoid, Alter, Adapt, and Accept—to reduce your stress and create a more peaceful environment for your baby. The techniques below can help you deal with stress by either changing the situation (Avoid and Alter) or changing your reaction (Adapt and Accept).

#### Change the Situation

**Avoid the stressor:** This means making changes to your environment to keep stress to a minimum. Are you spending a great deal of time with people who cause you stress (and therefore stress your baby)? Are you participating in activities and events that make you feel stressed out? Learn to say "no" and avoid people and situations that stress you. This is a time to change from being a "people pleaser" to thinking about pleasing and caring for you and your baby first.

**Alter the stressor:** If you cannot avoid the stressor, how can you change it? Can you modify your hours at work? Can you manage your time better? Can you move to a department with a lighter work load or can you work better hours during pregnancy? See how you can team up with coworkers, friends, and family to lighten your load, or do these activities with the people you love. When changing the stressor seems impossible, connect to your baby and make a determination to find a way to create even a small change.

### Change Your Reaction

**Adapt to the stressor:** How can you see the situation in a different way? Are you looking for the good in the situation or staying in a negative frame of mind? Talk about how the situation makes you feel with people you care about, such as your best friend, a counselor, or your spiritual support team. Think about how it would feel for your baby if you changed your reaction. Change how you see things and put the situation in perspective.

**Accept the stressor:** Sometimes it is impossible to change what is happening or the impact a stressor has on your life. In this case, you can choose your reaction to the stressor even if you cannot change it. Letting go of the need to control the situation can be a big step to reducing stress. When you embrace acceptance, you are no longer in a state of resistance, and this leads to a more peaceful internal state. An excellent affirmation for acceptance is, "I accept this situation in my life, and I trust that all things are working together for my highest good." You can also communicate to your baby that you are sorry that this situation has created stress but that you love your baby very much and want your baby to feel secure.

## Just Breathe

Another excellent way to reduce stress is to breathe deeply. In fact, many mothers feel that they become more mindful of their baby when practicing deep-breathing techniques. Now, you know how to breathe. Breathing is as much a part of your life as thinking. However, learning specific breathing techniques or "patterned breathing" (like those you might have seen on television where moms are breathing in a "hee, hee, hoo, hoo" pattern) will not significantly reduce stress. Patterned breath work causes you to use the "thinking" part of your brain. This keeps you from surrendering to your instinctual processes and can actually increase anxiety and inhibit the release of endorphins, your feel-good hormones.

The following breathing activities were created to help you become aware of how you breathe. Most people breathe in shallow, quick breaths as they breathe throughout the day. This is sometimes called *backward breathing*, and it is an indication of tension and stress in the body. A sign that you are breathing in this manner is that your chest moves more than your abdomen during inhalation and exhalation. The body works best when deep breathing is used, as it stimulates not only the lungs but also the diaphragm, pelvis, abdomen, and pineal gland (important for relaxation). This is the type of breathing that will benefit you and your baby throughout pregnancy and even in labor. If practiced regularly, deep breathing will become the normal pattern for your breath.

Breathing techniques like the following can significantly reduce your overall stress. Best of all, these techniques can be done anywhere, even at work, and they can help you feel more in touch with your baby.

## ACTIVITY: CLEANSING BREATH

Inhale deeply through the nose, pause slightly at the top of the breath, and then exhale slowly through the mouth. You can repeat as many times as it feels good.

This breath will fully oxygenate you and your baby when you experience a stressful moment. A cleansing breath can also help you move into a state of focus and relaxed attention. It is meant to cleanse the mind and release stress hormones from the body. ●

## ACTIVITY: BELLY BREATHING OR "DEEP BREATHING"

- Place your hands on your chest and inhale as you normally breathe. Notice how your lungs expand. Now place your hands on your diaphragm, just above your abdomen. If you do not notice your hands moving with your breath here, you are using shallow or backward breathing.

- Now inhale deeply into your abdomen, feeling your belly bulge out under your hands. As you exhale, notice how your hand moves inward toward your spine. Practice this deep breathing, trying to keep your exhale approximately twice as long as your inhale. Some people use a four/six count when first practicing deep breathing, inhaling for a count of four and exhaling for a count of six.

As you practice deep breathing, imagine your breath first filling your lungs, then your abdomen, then your pelvis, and then the rest of your body, all the way down to your toes. With your exhalation, pay attention to your breath as it leaves the body. Imagine breathing into the space where your baby lies, filling your baby with oxygen, and exhaling any tension that you or your baby may have. Feel your attachment to your baby as you breathe. ●

## ACTIVITY: DIAPHRAGMATIC BREATH WITH SIGH

For this breathing exercise, you'll need to practice the deep-breathing techniques mentioned prior, only add a sigh upon exhalation.

- Inhale deeply through the nose and exhale with a "haaaaa" sound. Sound is a wonderful way to release tension, stress, and even pain from the body. After practicing this diaphragmatic breath for several minutes, try tightening up all of the muscles in your face, hands, and legs and holding your breath for a count of eight.

- As you exhale with the "haaaaa" sound, allow all the tension you have just built up to be released. Do this several more times.

- Conclude this exercise by doing deep breathing with your hands on your abdomen, feeling the movement of your breath, and bringing your attention to your baby. This breath work is particularly helpful to release tension in the body after a stressful encounter, and when practiced can create a sense of safety for your baby. ●

## ACTIVITY: THREE-PART BREATHING

- Practice deep-breathing techniques for several minutes. As you deeply breathe, tune in to your connection to your baby. With your next breath, draw your breath first into your belly as much as you can, then into your diaphragm, and finally, with the last bit of breath, inhale deeply into the lungs. Use your hands and feel your belly bulge, then your rib cage, and finally your upper chest.

- As you exhale, allow your breath to move out of your upper chest first, then your rib cage, and finally your abdomen. This breathing exercise takes some time to master. It is an excellent way to rid yourself of tension and bring awareness into your breathing. ●

The body scan is a technique used to release tension from the muscles in the body and encourage deep relaxation. It is often practiced while lying down.

- Practice your deep-breathing techniques for several minutes. When you feel calm and centered, continue deep breathing and place your focus on your head. Notice any tension around or between your eyes, in your jaw line, or in your tongue. Let go of any tension you feel here. Slowly move your attention down the body. Notice your neck muscles, shoulders, arms, and hands. Soften these areas of the body and feel the tension melting away.
- Next, bring your awareness to your chest, abdomen, and your low back. Release any tightness in these areas. Then work your way down through your buttocks, thighs, and calves, all the way down through your feet. When you notice tension, bring your awareness to that area and consciously focus on releasing the tension with your breath. ●

## Smile and Yawn

Smiling and yawning are also excellent stress relievers. What could be easier than curling the edges of your lips upwards and bursting into a smile or taking in a deep breath and yawning? It may sound strange, but these two behaviors have been found to have profound effects on stress reduction and mood enhancement, which you now know benefits your baby and attachment pregnancy too!

The benefits of smiling include:

- People are kinder and gentler to you
- It calms you down
- It stabilizes your mood and the mood of those around you

- It creates a feeling of security and happiness
- You feel more sympathetic to those around you
- Smiling is contagious (scientific fact!)
- Smiling sends positive thought molecules to your baby

All of these things create a healthier pregnancy and emotional environment for you, which is better for your baby.

It sounds strange, but yawning also has enormous health benefits. Researchers have found that yawning can calm the mind in less than a minute. Practice yawning at least twelve to fifteen times in a row, pausing for a few seconds between each yawn for optimal benefit. If you find it challenging, just "fake yawn" until real yawning begins. Yawning stimulates a part of the brain called the precuneous, which is partly responsible for feelings of empathy, consciousness, and self-awareness. These all contribute to the motherbaby bond. Yawning helps you reset and stabilize your mind. So give it a go, sit back, relax, and yawn!

There are many benefits of yawning, all of which are good for mother and baby. Yawning:

- Reduces anxiety
- Increases empathy
- Improves memory retrieval
- Optimizes your metabolism
- Increases your sense of compassion
- Heightens your state of awareness
- Helps you sleep better
- Lowers stress
- Relaxes the body

When you incorporate the simple acts of smiling and yawning into your daily stress-reduction routine, you will not only get the stress-reduction benefits so important to attachment pregnancy, you will receive all of the benefits just mentioned.

## Focus on Your Heart Space

Another way to reduce stress is to focus not only on your breath, but the space around your heart (heart space), which we discussed briefly in Chapter 4. This allows you to root yourself more deeply in the present and practice Be-ing. Many cultures around the world have recognized the importance of the heart for optimal emotional and physical health: Yogic traditions teach about the heart chakra as the seat of balance and consciousness, and religious traditions such as Christianity, Judaism, and Islam also refer to the importance of connecting to the heart for emotional clarity. The researchers at the Institute of HeartMath have found a variety of ways that simply focusing on the energy of the heart can help reduce stress, including . . .

### The Balance Hormone

Researchers have found that your heart actually "thinks," as it is made up of neural tissue like the brain. It has a separate neurosystem from the brain and does not really even need the brain to function. The heart actually communicates to the brain, and the brain responds. Your heart reads the environment around you, which can move you into a stress response. Your awareness of environment, through the act of observing, will help you manage your stress level. The heart also produces its own hormone, ANF, which is known as "the balance hormone." This hormone helps reduce the effects of stress by helping to control your blood pressure.

### Heart Rhythms

As we discussed in Chapter 4, your heart has an electromagnetic field, which extends out at least eight feet beyond your body and actually communicates with the electromagnetic fields of other people's hearts. Your heart speaks to the hearts of those around you. This is one reason why you may feel uncomfortable when you are near someone who is in a completely different emotional state than you. That person's heart rhythm feels uncomfortable to you because it is out of sync with your heart rhythm. The longer you are around another person, the more likely it is that your heart rhythms will sync. You will literally feel their stress or their happiness based on their heart resonance, as the heart's magnetic energy changes depending on the individual's emotional state. Remember that your heart significantly affects your baby's heart, which is another reason why you should carefully select those who are around you and your baby. They can impact your and your baby's emotional state and stress level. Your heart rate directly affects the flow of blood and nourishment to your baby via the placenta. A healthy heart pattern and rhythm means a healthy blood flow to your baby. Blood flow to your baby nourishes her, oxygenates her, and removes toxins from her environment.

The heart is the seat of your emotional quotient, or EQ, and is constantly communicating with the emotional centers in your brain. When your heart is out of balance due to negative emotions (anxiety, anger, and fear), it creates a disorderly beat and rhythm called *incoherence*. Positive emotions, such as love, appreciation, and care, create order and harmony in the heart's rhythm, which helps optimize health. This is called a *coherent heart pattern*. These positive emotions are associated with increased immunity, reduced stress hormones, and hormonal balance—all key factors for an attachment pregnancy. The bottom line is that, when you surround yourself with positive people, you—and your baby—will feel their positive emotions and benefit from that positivity!

### Your Baby's Heart and Brain Development

Your baby's heart develops long before her brain does, and the emotional regions of the brain develop before the intellectual parts of the brain do. You are first communicating intuitively with your baby's heart through entrainment early in pregnancy. Your baby is first an emotional, feeling person before she is a thinking person. Her feelings make up her world and all that she knows of the world. Pregnancy is the time when you will have the greatest impact on her emotional health.

During pregnancy your baby's brain develops based on *your* heart and brain-wave patterns. The amygdala, the emotional center of your baby's brain, develops according to the state of coherence or incoherence in your body. If your heart and brain are in a state of coherence during pregnancy (experiencing states of love, appreciation, and care), your baby's brain develops to seek out peaceful situations (coherence) for the rest of her life. If your heart and brain are in a state of incoherence during pregnancy (experiencing anxiety, anger, and fear), then your baby's brain develops to seek out chaos to feel "normal." Humans always want to feel "at home" and will search out situations, people, and environments that help them feel normal even if that norm is unhealthy, so how you feel during your pregnancy will impact how your child navigates the rest of her life—who she develops relationships with and situations she will seek out. So help design your baby's brain to look for peace and happiness by cultivating these things in your own life during pregnancy.

### Use Your Heart to Reduce Stress

To use your heart intelligence to reduce stress, start by becoming mindful of your thoughts, using deep-breathing techniques, and focusing your awareness on your heart center. Think about something that makes you happy, someone you love, or something that you appreciate and begin moving into a state of gratitude. The researchers at the Institute of HeartMath have designed specific techniques for maximizing your heart's intelligence. Check them out by visiting their website: *www.heartmath.org.*

## Creativity

As mentioned, this trimester is a time to be present and nurture the connection between you and your baby. A great way for you to do this is by tapping into the creative flow that pregnancy offers. You may find that you feel especially artistic and expressive during your pregnancy. Additionally, taking time to express your creativity can significantly help with stress reduction. One of the reasons you become so creative is because pregnancy and mothering is a right-brained activity.

The right side of the brain is associated with feeling and learns with heart or body knowledge, and the left side of the brain is associated with thinking and learns with head knowledge. The right hemisphere of the brain is known for regulating empathy, trust, self-awareness, emotion, and stress; it is the creative, holistic part of your brain. As your right brain hemisphere begins to become more primary during pregnancy and early mothering, you'll find yourself more attracted to artistic activities, more drawn to creative expression. The act of mothering is intuitive, spontaneous, and creative, which means that your right brain hemisphere is engaged for better mothering. In fact, your baby will primarily be functioning from her right brain hemisphere in the womb and for the first three years of her life, which puts you and your baby more in tune with one another and promotes attachment.

This discovery is one that can be enormously helpful to you in pregnancy. Tuning in to your inner self can be a powerful way to discover your true feelings, dreams, hopes, and even your fears and worries. Connecting to this part of you can help you work through some of these fears, which can enhance the motherbaby bond. It can also better prepare you for your baby's birth and for being the best mother you can be. You may not feel that you have time to be creative or that it is unimportant compared to your long to-do list; however, allowing time for creative expression enhances an attachment pregnancy. So make a date with your baby and put creative playtime on your calendar several times a week during pregnancy.

### Express Your Creativity

There are many ways you can express your creativity. You can paint, draw, journal, knit, work with clay, and do crafting activities—even cooking can be creative expression. Find something that helps you relax and express yourself. One particularly helpful creative expression for pregnancy is journaling, as it helps you become more connected to your deepest feelings and needs. Gather up some creative tools that you need, such as beautiful paper or a journal and your favorite-color pen. This is your artwork and should reflect the inner you, so feel free to use what feels good. Write about your feelings and thoughts often, and spend some time reflecting on what you have written. Keep your journal private so that you can be open and honest with yourself. You instinctively know what you really need, and if you journal regularly, these needs will be revealed through your writing.

Here are some ideas for sentence stems to start journaling:

- What I already know about my baby is . . .
- What excites me the most about becoming a mother is . . .
- What scares me the most during this pregnancy is . . .
- What I am finding out about myself during this pregnancy is . . .
- What I need today is . . .
- How I am going about getting my needs met during pregnancy is . . .
- What I am learning about my relationship with my partner during this pregnancy is . . .
- What I want to give my baby is . . .

While you may or may not have previously felt creative in your former, nonpregnant life, the mere fact that you are pregnant has opened up the pathways in your brain to support being creative. Remember that when you are expressing yourself creatively, you are releasing beneficial hormones that support your attachment pregnancy. Take advantage of this ability now.

> "Instead of wishing away nine months of pregnancy, I'd have cherished every moment, realizing that the wonderment growing inside me was the only chance in life to assist God in a miracle."
>
> ~Erma Bombeck, American Humorist, Columnist, and Author

### ACTIVITY: WRITE A LOVE LETTER TO YOUR BABY

A great way to tap into your creative mind during pregnancy and to intensify your bond with your baby is to write a love letter to your baby. The best way to write a letter that truly taps into your heart space is to first use the guidelines for Conscious Attachment discussed in Chapter 4. Write your letter as if you are talking directly to your baby. Here are some suggestions to get your creative juices flowing:

- Your wishes and dreams for your baby
- Things you want to show/do with your baby someday
- How you feel about your baby
- What you already know about your baby
- Share with your baby news about the family's excitement for her arrival
- Share positive or loving comments that family and friends have said about the baby

Once you have finished your letter, date it, seal it, and save it for a future keepsake. ●

Be gentle and kind to yourself, and follow your instincts to connect with your inner wisdom for an attachment pregnancy. Remember, it is impossible to live a stress-free life. You can, however, live a life of gratitude and appreciation and learn how to manage the stressful events of life. You choose how you react to the events in your life. These tools will benefit your pregnancy, your bond with your baby, your family, and your ability to parent for the rest of your life.

# CHAPTER SUMMARY

Reducing stress is the key to a happier, healthier pregnancy and baby. A commitment to stress reduction is essential to an attachment pregnancy. Remember:

- Your body experiences two types of stress: eustress (positive stress) and distress (negative stress). Distress can put a pregnant woman into a state of "tend or befriend," which can prevent you from practicing self-care and attachment.

- Acute or short-term stress is not harmful to your baby. Chronic or persistent stress, however, can negatively impact your pregnancy and the long-term health of your baby.

- You have the power to reduce your stress during pregnancy. There are simple ways to reduce stress ranging from deep breathing, to physical activity, to smiling.

- You can use the four As of stress reduction—Avoid, Alter, Adapt, and Accept—to reduce your stress and create a more peaceful environment for your baby.

- Deep breathing is an excellent way to practice stress reduction. Try the cleansing breath, belly breathing, diaphragmatic breathing with a sigh, three-part breathing, or the body scan with deep breathing.

- Smiling and yawning can also reduce stress and enhance your mood, which deepens the motherbaby bond.

- Your heart communicates via an electromagnetic field with those around you and, most significantly, with your baby. This heart-to-heart communication also directs the development of your baby's brain. Your positive emotions can shape your baby's brain in an optimal way.

- To use your heart intelligence to reduce stress, become mindful of your thoughts, use deep-breathing techniques, and focus your awareness on your heart center.

- Pregnancy is intuitive, spontaneous, and creative, which means that your right brain hemisphere is engaged for better mothering and is primed for attachment. Allow time for creative expression to enhance your attachment pregnancy.

# CHAPTER 8

# The Physical Bond

> "Did you ever stop to taste a carrot? Not just eat it, but taste it? You can't taste the beauty and energy of the earth in a Twinkie."
>
> ~Astrid Alauda, Philosopher

Your physical health significantly impacts how you feel during pregnancy and therefore affects your ability to bond with your baby, which means there is no time like pregnancy to start embracing healthy decisions regarding your body. Making healthy choices in Conscious Agreement, such as actively choosing a crisp, ripe apple over greasy chips for a snack, allows you to begin to see each moment as an opportunity for vitality, instead of a burden that you are saddled with. Choosing actions that support a healthy pregnancy lifestyle create a body that is better able to support your baby, but it's important to realize that health in pregnancy comes from more than just what you eat, drink, and do for exercise. It is also impacted by how you feel about your body and how you care for it; making choices that positively benefit your and your baby's health is proactive parenting at its best. Remember that during pregnancy nutrition is a partnership. Your deep attachment to your baby will help guide you toward making better choices. What choices can you make? How can you strengthen that physical bond with your baby? Read on . . .

## Make Choices You Feel Good About

How you feel about the choices you make during your pregnancy is perhaps more important than the choices themselves. Your body is an expression of your internal, emotional world. This emotional state directly affects the health of your developing baby and the health of your pregnancy. Your baby is always aware of how you are feeling about the choices you make. When you make healthy choices in a positive state of mind, your baby develops in a safe and secure environment and feels your positivity, which promotes attachment. When you make choices that cause you to feel resentment and guilt, your baby's development is hindered and the motherbaby bond is diminished. Your observation of the choices you make changes the physical health of you and your baby and affects your attachment to your baby. When you consciously make healthy choices, you express your love for your baby. The attachment pregnancy flourishes when gratitude and mindfulness are at the core of health decisions.

## Nutrition

Changing your diet and eating healthy can seem like an overwhelming task, but the reality is that the food you eat impacts pregnancy health, including the hormones your body releases. For example, when you eat food high in tryptophan, such as pumpkin seeds, your brain releases more seratonin. (You will learn more about specific hormones and food choices in Part 4.) Additionally, your nutrition choices change the pH of your body, which affects every organ system in your body. When your body is acidic instead of alkaline, it sets the stage for disease, such as cancer, for you and your baby. Most mothers today consume far too many acidic foods, such as sodas, dairy products, meat products, and processed foods. The best choice is to eat clean, vibrant, naturally colorful foods in as much variety as you can. The following tips can be easily incorporated into your life and will keep you on the right path toward a healthy attachment pregnancy.

## Practice Healthy Weight Gain

Every woman will find that her body needs to gain a different amount of weight during pregnancy, though the suggested weight gain is between 25 and 35 pounds. As long as you focus on eating a variety of healthy, nourishing foods like those discussed later on in this chapter, exercise your body daily, and practice daily breathing activities, your body should be guided to gain the appropriate amount of weight. You may not realize this, but pregnancy should not be a time for dieting *or* overindulging on a regular basis. Surprisingly, your body only needs about an extra 300 calories a day to grow and adequately nourish your baby, and those 300 calories should be nutrient-dense. A 200-calorie cookie and a 200-calorie fresh fruit salad are not equal choices during pregnancy; choose the food options that will deliver the most nutrition to you and your baby. Keep Conscious Agreement and Conscious Attachment in mind when it is time to nourish your body and baby; these techniques will help keep you in balance and prevent eating extremes. If you're concerned about gaining weight during your pregnancy, it's important to realize that this is a natural part of the process and that the weight you're gaining is there for a reason. Also, this isn't weight that's going right to your hips, thighs, or tummy. The following is a guide to show you the average weight gain of different body parts during pregnancy:

| WEIGHT GAIN CHART | |
|---|---|
| *Body Part* | *Pounds* |
| Blood Volume | 3 pounds |
| Breast Tissue | 2 pounds |
| Uterus | 2 pounds |
| Baby | 6.5 - 9 pounds |
| Placenta | 1.5 pounds |
| Amniotic Fluid | 2 pounds |
| Fat and Protein | 7 pounds |
| Water | 4 pounds |

Instead of obsessing about what the scale says, focus your loving awareness on what you are eating and how it is contributing to the healthy growth of your child. This is another way to focus on your baby, which increases attachment.

## Be Mindful

Practice mindfulness when you eat. This means listening to your actual hunger cravings, paying attention to how things really taste, and recognizing when you actually feel full. Using mindfulness for nutrition in pregnancy has been proven to reduce emotional eating, minimize overeating, and encourage healthier choices. Just as your heart has neural tissue and "thinks" on its own, so does your digestive system. Your gut sends a message to your brain based on what you eat, which helps control your mood, your cravings, and even your personality. For example, when you continuously eat foods that are high in sugar, this creates a habitual craving within your brain. Additionally, it changes your blood sugar levels, which affect your moods. When you consistently are experiencing moodiness, this negatively affects your personality. This chain of events can happen with many types of processed foods as well. Remember, your nutrition choices impact your baby's moods, future food cravings, disease risk, and personality. When you eat healthy foods, you reduce your baby's risk of diabetes, heart disease, and obesity and strengthen your attachment pregnancy. How does nutrition affect the motherbaby bond in attachment pregnancy? When you nourish yourself mindfully, you show love for yourself and your baby, and your baby feels that love in the womb.

## Eat Clean and Natural

During your attachment pregnancy, it's important to remember that whatever you eat is what your baby eats too, so choose wisely! Try to eat foods that are organic, natural, and not processed; they allow your body to make maximal use of the vitamins, minerals, phytoestrogens, fats, and other properties in the foods. Often, organic and minimally processed foods are more nutrient-dense in the properties your pregnant body needs. Unfortunately, typical, mass-produced vegetables contain chemicals, waxes, and pesticides that can affect your developing baby and even your milk when you are breastfeeding. Foods that have been exposed to these harmful agents can potentially affect your baby's genes and gene expression, depending on the type of agent and the amount of the exposure. Certain agents can even transfer into breastmilk, exposing your baby in that way. Keep in mind though, that no matter what your diet is, breastmilk is always superior in nutrition over artificial milk (infant formula). Keep the following advice in mind:

- When choosing meat and dairy products, which can be important sources of protein for pregnancy, try to choose pasture-raised animals that have not been exposed to growth hormones.
- Cage-free poultry and eggs have higher amounts of omega fatty acids, which are critical for your developing baby. Omega fatty acids are called *essential* fatty acids because they are essential to

healthy development of your baby's brain, eyes, skin, and other organs.

- Choose fish that are less likely to be laden with mercury, such as sardines, anchovies, wild salmon, and flounder. Eating fish rich in omega fatty acids will also help you think better! Fish to avoid or eat in very limited quantities include any farm-raised fish (such as tilapia), shark, swordfish, king mackerel, and yes, tuna.

- Avoid processed foods whenever possible. You are actually creating your baby's cravings for certain foods and flavors during pregnancy, including your baby's drive to consume fat, sugar, and salt. All processed foods are developed after much research and testing to create the most addictive combination of fat, sugar, and salt that will encourage the highest consumption. The levels of salt, sugar, and fat found in processed foods are not found in nature, and the more you eat them, the more you prewire your baby's brain to desire unhealthy foods. In addition, foods with trans fats should be avoided as often as possible.

- Eat fresh foods that will rot quickly. These foods are not filled with preservatives and trans fats. All packaged and fast foods are loaded with preservatives (including added salt, fat, and sugar) and are unlikely to rot anytime soon. Choose wisely, and more often than not, choose clean and natural.

## Enjoy Healthy Oils

Yes, it's true, many oils and fats are good for you, especially during pregnancy. The latest USDA food guide, called MyPlate, encourages pregnant women to include healthy oils in their diets. Though oils should be eaten in Conscious Agreement, they are still part of a healthy pregnancy diet. Many of the cooking oils on the grocery store shelves have been processed and are often rancid. You can find fresh, higher-quality cooking oils at health food stores or places that specialize in freshly pressed oils, like specialty oil shops and online stores. The best oils for cooking are extra virgin olive oil, avocado oil, coconut oil, ghee (clarified butter), organic butter, peanut oil, and high oleic sunflower and safflower oil. Oils such as low-grade olive oil (often called light olive oil), grapeseed oil, flaxseed oil, and walnut oil are best for tossing on salads and drizzling over veggies, because the chemical makeup of these oils changes when they're exposed to high heat, and they lose their health benefits.

Most oils should be kept only a couple of months and should be stored in dark bottles in a cool place. Only buy what you need! Buy organic, as most pesticides are fat-soluble, which means pesticides can accumulate in high quantities in pressed oils. One of the best things you can do to improve your and your baby's health is to throw away any and all margarine in your refrigerator. If you need buttery flavor, use real butter or use ghee (found in most health food stores)—just use small amounts. The hydrogenated oils (trans fats) in margarine are bad for your growing baby's brain and neural system development.

Even better than drizzling foods with healthy oils is to eat the natural source—eat a nut, crack open a coconut, snack on seeds, eat an olive! Additional important sources of healthy fats are avocados, flax seeds, and wild-caught, small fish or bottom-dwelling fish (anchovies, flounder, sardines, and salmon). But no matter how you eat these oils, your baby's brain will be 60 percent fat by weight, so supply her with healthy brain-building fats!

## Nosh on Veggies!

Most vegetables are alkaline foods, and this supports a healthy environment for pregnancy. If you are in the early weeks of pregnancy, focus on alkaline-rich foods, not acidic foods (like meats and dairy). Examples of alkaline foods include dark, leafy vegetables, almonds, asparagus, and mangoes. You can find many alkaline food charts with a quick web search. Eat veggies with deep, rich colors, because they have more micronutrients and phytochemicals that will help protect your baby from free radicals, which damage cells. The darker, more colorful varieties are also more flavorful, which will only encourage you to eat more of them!

## Don't Forget Your Vitamins and Minerals!

Vitamins and minerals that you obtain from the foods you eat are essential to your developing baby. Your baby needs this nutrition to effectively grow organs. You are the only source of vitamins and minerals that your baby has, so your nutrition is key. Excellent sources for vitamins and minerals are juicy fruits and vegetables like apples, mangoes, raspberries, and blueberries. If fresh fruits are not readily available, try flash-frozen fruits as a great substitute. Or try a berry-and-Greek-yogurt smoothie for a mid-morning snack instead of relying on a candy bar for energy. It will deliver great nutrition and satisfy your sweet tooth! Remember, your health is a bond that you and your baby share.

### Take a Supplement

If you manage to eat a varied and nutritionally balanced diet, there is no need to use a supplement. However, most mothers have days they want to order French fries, forget to pack a plum in their lunch sack, or choose to snack on chips instead of broccoli, so complementing your diet with a multivitamin supplement is a good idea for most pregnant women. Zinc, selenium, and vitamins A, C, E, and B complex—including folic acid, which is particularly important during the first trimester, when your baby's neural system is developing—are important to pregnancy. Each of these vitamins and minerals has a specific property that helps the healthy development of your baby to progress. Find a whole food vitamin that contains these nutrients.

Whole food vitamins, as opposed to synthetic vitamins (most over-the-counter vitamins), are produced from real food, not created from chemicals in a lab. Your body knows how to process whole food vitamins and get the most out of the nutrients they contain. Whole food vitamins contain vitamins and minerals in a natural food state, meaning they are found with companion nutrients that help your body digest them better. They are also less likely to cause nausea and stomach upset. On the other hand, synthetic vitamins can contain toxins that can accumulate in your body, so go natural! Many doctors unknowingly offer prescriptions for prenatal synthetic vitamins because they are unaware of the potential side effects and physical discomforts they cause, such as constipation and increased nausea.

Check with your care provider about which whole food vitamin alternatives he or she might suggest (or talk to a nutritionist or natural healthcare provider who specializes in pregnancy).

## Avoid No-Value Foods

No-value foods include sugar, white flour, and white rice, which turn quickly into simple carbohydrates that do nothing to enhance your and your baby's health. White sugar also elevates stress hormones, something you now know you want to avoid in pregnancy. If you must sweeten your food, avoid *all* chemical sweeteners, such as aspartame, saccharine, and sucralose. Long-term studies have not shown these chemical additives to be safe for pregnancy, so it's best to avoid them. Better options are maple sugar, molasses, and honey.

When you begin to replace white flour products with whole grain alternatives, you will begin to see how delicious real grains are. Better alternatives for no-value grains are barley, oatmeal, buckwheat, quinoa, amaranth, brown rice, and wild rice. These are all delicious alternatives to white starches, and they are filled with vitamins. Make a double or triple batch of healthy grains when you cook them so you can store the extra and have some on hand for easy sides and salad mixes throughout the week.

To make sure you're eating foods full of the nutrients you need during your pregnancy, shop the perimeter of the grocery store, as well as the tops and bottoms of the store racks (instead of the middle, eye-level rack) where healthier, nonprocessed foods tend to be. Grocery stores tend to place their high-cost, superprocessed foods near the entry and in the center of the store, knowing that will entice you to purchase these items.

## Exercise and Movement

In addition to eating well, exercise and movement are part of an attachment pregnancy. The simple act of moving sends a nourishing blood flow throughout your body, to all of your organs, and to your growing baby. It can also remove stress hormones from your body, which creates a more peaceful environment for your baby. It also lubricates your joints, which can alleviate many aches and pains as your pregnancy progresses. Exercise is also a natural antidepressant and, when depression is decreased, attachment is increased. To get these benefits, commit to some sort of body movement for at least thirty minutes a day. Whether it is a walk, yoga, a hike, dancing, swimming, or a prenatal exercise class, just move! Your exercise time during pregnancy is a perfect opportunity for one-on-one bonding time with your baby.

### Prenatal Yoga

Prenatal yoga is a wonderful way to connect your body, mind, spirit, and baby. Yoga allows you to practice mindfulness and begin to cultivate a nonjudgmental, accepting attitude about your body and your life. As your body grows with pregnancy, yoga helps you develop a love and acceptance of your changing body, and prenatal yoga has also been shown to increase mobility; improve circulation; reduce certain pregnancy discomforts such as backache, heartburn, and sciatica; reduce blood pressure; elevate your mood; and improve sleep. Mothers report being better able to tune in to their babies during and just after the practice of yoga, which deepens their bond. Prenatal yoga has also been associated with reduced stress, reduced preterm delivery, healthy birth weights, and fewer birth complications.

The general goals of prenatal yoga are to:

- Enhance body awareness as changes of pregnancy occur
- Help alleviate certain physical discomforts, such as backache
- Bond deeply with the baby (deepen attachment pregnancy)
- Evoke deep relaxation states
- Develop flexibility, strength, balance, and agility
- Nurture community
- Learn to cope with stress in healthy ways
- Develop comfort measures to cope with labor and birth

Prenatal yoga can help you as an expectant mother connect your body, mind, and spirit. This ancient practice allows you to connect to your baby and your body as it begins to transform. Yoga invites you into a world of balance, peace, and mindfulness. If possible, try and find a class where you can meet other moms and have an experienced yoga teacher help usher you through your pregnancy.

But while mothers in relatively any stage of fitness can participate in a prenatal yoga class and find many benefits, there are certain complications in later stages of pregnancy that are considered contraindications for the practice. They include ruptured membranes, persistent bleeding, placenta previa, pre-eclampsia or toxemia, early cervical dilation, and uncontrolled cardiovascular disease. In the event that you experience any of these symptoms, you will want to talk to your healthcare provider before continuing your yoga practice. It's actually a good idea to always check with your health-care provider before initiating any new form of exercise.

Your body is communicating with you throughout your pregnancy. Take time to listen in and pay attention to the needs of your body and your baby. Ultimately, it will lead to a healthier attachment pregnancy.

# CHAPTER SUMMARY

Your physical health significantly impacts how you feel during pregnancy and therefore affects your ability to bond with your baby. Taking a mindful approach to your physical wellness contributes to mind, body, and spirit health for you and your baby during attachment pregnancy. Remember:

- The food you eat impacts pregnancy health, including the hormones your body releases. The best choices for you and your baby are to eat clean, vibrant, naturally colorful foods in as much variety as you can.

- Use Conscious Agreement and Conscious Attachment when it is time to nourish your body and baby; these techniques will help keep you in balance and prevent eating extremes.

- Practice being mindful when you eat, meaning you listen to your actual hunger cravings, pay attention to how things really taste, and recognize when you actually feel full.

- Eating foods that are organic, natural, and not processed allows your body to make maximal use of the properties in the foods.

- Though oils should be consumed consciously, they are still part of a healthy pregnancy diet.

- Eat veggies with deep, rich colors, because they have more micronutrients and phytochemicals that will help protect your baby from free radicals, which damage cells.

- Most women should take whole food vitamins during pregnancy, which contain vitamins and minerals in a natural food state.

- Excellent sources for vitamins and minerals are juicy fruits and vegetables. Typically, the deeper the color of a fruit or vegetable, the more nutrients and antioxidants it contains.

- Avoid no-value foods, including sugar, white flour, and white rice, which turn quickly into simple carbohydrates that do nothing to enhance your or your baby's health.

- Exercise and movement are part of an attachment pregnancy, as they can reduce stress, improve blood flow, alleviate certain pregnancy discomforts, and reduce depression. Prenatal yoga, in particular, is a wonderful way to connect your body, mind, spirit, and baby.

# CHAPTER 9

# Your Relationships and Your Baby

> "Call it a clan, call it a network, call it a tribe, call it a family. Whatever you call it, whoever you are, you need one."
> ~Elizabeth Jane Howard, Novelist

Your family, your friends, your coworkers, your spiritual support team, and your healthcare team will all be part of your and your baby's support system. Even as early as the first trimester, your relationships will impact your developing baby, because your relationships impact your belief systems and your stress level. Now is the time to focus on your most supportive relationships and observe your relationships with friends and family, your community, and your source/higher power. Who in your life provides you with the support, love, and connection that will ultimately lead to a supported pregnancy and a deeper bond with your baby? In this chapter, you will find out why these relationships are so important during the first trimester of an attachment pregnancy.

## Why During Pregnancy?

Pregnancy is an opportunity to observe the impact that your important relationships have on your life, and ultimately the bond between you and your baby. You can consciously choose to create a deeper bond with those who positively impact you, or you can choose to limit your relationships with those that have a negative impact on you, depending on how you feel when you are with them. Relationships begin when you are growing inside your own mother, and continue to form in the early years of your life. These relationships become embedded in your subconscious. It is important to be aware of this as you are growing and nurturing your child during your pregnancy.

As we discussed in Chapter 5, your baby's experiences of your relationships in utero teach her about trust and safety in her world. Studies show that babies have a physical and emotional reaction to the mother's relationships prior to being born. In fact, babies in utero have been seen on ultrasound crying and reacting in fear to simulated fights between parents. When a baby continuously experiences a mother's negative emotional reaction to someone in her life, the baby actually learns to withdraw. She learns not to "trust" this relationship and therefore does not have a safe haven with her mother. When you protect yourself and your baby by consciously choosing to engage in relationships that support the two of you, your baby will feel protected, safe, and secure. This ensures attachment and strengthens the motherbaby bond.

The first trimester is a perfect time for you to start observing your relationships and defining what they mean to you and your future family. It will take time for you to make changes in your relationships; they won't happen overnight. This period of development is the foundation for your baby's emotional health, so starting early to create your healthy community of relationships is important. There is a reason pregnancy takes nine full months, as it gives you the opportunity to observe what needs to change and take the actions necessary to support what you and your baby need.

## Your Family

Even though you do not get to choose your family, you do get to choose the relationship that you have with your family. This becomes even more important when you are expecting a baby, because these relationships will not only affect your life but will affect the health of your growing baby and your ability to feel a sense of connection to your baby. When observing your relationships with your extended family, it is common to believe that there is nothing that you can do about those relationships that feel unsupportive. You may think that you must tolerate these unsupportive relationships, or that you have no control over them because they are with family members. Remember that, as we discussed in Chapter 5, you are always in control of your relationship boundaries. Even if you have wonderful relationships with your family members, you may still need to create some boundaries.

Consider: how do you want your child to begin her relationships with your extended family? It all starts with how you see your family now, and how you feel about each family member. Your perceptions of your relationships become your child's perceptions. The current health of your family is the basis for the health of the family you are creating. Take some time in the next few days to really consider this.

> **"If you think you are so enlightened, go spend a week with your parents."**
>
> ~Ram Dass, Contemporary Spiritual Teacher
> and Author of *Be Here Now*

Are your family relationships generally gratifying, loving, and nurturing? Do they support an attachment pregnancy? If so, you should focus on spending more time and energy on these relationships. Are your relationships a source of anger, anxiety, and stress? Is it time to start healing and opening yourself up to forgiveness? Do you need to limit contact with these individuals? In emotionally/

physically abusive situations, you may need to completely end your exposure to certain individuals in order to create healthy and safe boundaries for you and your baby.

## Forgiveness

Regardless of any boundaries you decide to create, there are often lingering emotions and past experiences that can be healed by forgiveness. Forgiveness is about freeing yourself from the bondage of negative emotions you feel toward someone; forgiveness is not about absolution of guilt. Choosing to forgive does not change the past; rather, it frees you from the negative emotions of past events. It puts the power back in your court; no longer will the person or event hold power over you. A little forgiveness can go a long way, and it can help you to forge a healthier connection with the individual in question. Wouldn't you prefer for your child to have deep, loving, healthy, and happy connections in her life? Wouldn't you prefer for your baby to see you as her safe haven?

> **"To forgive is to set a prisoner free and discover that the prisoner was you."**
> ~Lewis B. Smedes, Renowned Christian Author and Theologian

For those family members (and, really, anyone in your life) that cause you to feel stress and anxiety, it is important to change your mind in order to change the way you feel about those people. It is not enough to simply acknowledge a negative emotion that you feel about someone close to you. These emotions are still connected to your baby. Additionally, when you are harboring negative emotions, such as anger, hatred, and resentment, it becomes impossible to be in the peaceful and loving state that optimizes bonding. To experience an attachment pregnancy, you must begin to see the relationship in a new light. To begin to do so, try this activity:

Sit for a moment, close your eyes, begin your deep breathing, and bring a vision of the person whom you feel negative emotion for into your awareness. Acknowledge the feelings you harbor for this person. Notice how those emotions feel in your body. Notice how your body and your baby react. Does it feel good? If not, note that your baby also feels these uncomfortable sensations. Your baby is first a feeling human and only later becomes a thinking human, so every emotion you feel becomes your child's world. Are you ready to change these negative emotions?

Take a deep breath. Envision that same person, and this time see him or her surrounded with light. Offer unrestricted love to this person. Pick out something that you feel grateful for in this relationship or as a result of this relationship, no matter how small. Focus on that feeling of gratitude. If it is impossible to feel gratitude, ask for help from your source. Ask, "Please help me see this person, this situation, in a more loving, peaceful way."

Wait a few moments. If you still feel anxiety, just focus on your heart center, breathe, and stay in the space of gratitude you have created for this person. Practice this technique every day and you will begin to see your relationship to this person change. It is not your family that causes you anxiety. It is how you *see* your family that causes your reaction. The boundaries that you create around your family and how you react to them are what cause the anxiety and stress that you experience. The boundaries that you develop, or lack thereof, can either strengthen or weaken the motherbaby bond. ●

## Key Concepts for Dealing with Your Family

The following suggestions can help you develop a stronger and more peaceful relationship with your family during pregnancy. While you can't change your family, you can change how you see your family and how you react to them.

- Your relationships with your family will change when you stop reacting to your own subconscious programming. Stop, look, and listen. How do you feel about this person when you place him or her in your heart space? Does it change things for you?
- You have no control over other people's actions. You cannot change your family. Wishing things will change is wasted energy. You can only change your response to them and how you see the situation.
- Let go of the desire to have your relationship with your family look a certain way. Instead, accept the way things are and find ways to be grateful for what those relationships bring to you and your growing baby.

The more that you begin to observe and reframe your relationship with your family during attachment pregnancy, the deeper the bond to your baby will become.

## The Importance of Friends

Humans need each other. Research shows that people who are part of a social network live longer and are more likely to survive life-threatening diseases. People who have a close circle of friends are more secure and have a greater sense of well-being. Remember that when you feel secure, so does your baby. It's easier to navigate through pregnancy's many choices when you know you and your baby are being supported.

Studies show that when you have secure and attached friendships, you are better able to create intimacy and secure additional attached relationships. Your ability to bond with others will help you to securely bond with your baby. When you focus on friendships where you can engage in a high level of trust, sharing, and hope, it creates a higher level of personal satisfaction and security. These qualities enhance the motherbaby bond. Simple ways to nourish friendships during pregnancy:

- When reaching out to friends, put an actual date on the calendar instead of saying, "Let's get together soon."
- Remember that e-mailing, Facebooking, and texting are not substitutions for in-person, heart-to-heart connecting. In fact, studies show that impersonal communication like social media does not elevate important pregnancy hormones, such as oxytocin.
- Make chore or errand time a time that you can gather with your friends. For example, go shopping for your baby registry with a friend instead of by yourself.
- Don't wait to see your friends until the end of the day, as pregnancy tends to make you tired in the evenings. Plan lunch or breakfast with your friends.
- Why exercise alone? Ask your friends to join you. You will receive all of the benefits of exercise *and* friendship.

Staying connected with your friends does take a certain amount of effort and energy; however, the positive feelings that you share with your friends contribute to your attachment pregnancy and are worth the effort.

## Other Expectant Mothers

Connecting with other expectant mothers during pregnancy is a wonderful way to fully come into motherhood. There are a variety of classes designed for expectant women, such as pregnancy exercise classes, prenatal yoga classes, childbirth classes, breastfeeding classes, and other types of support groups. By attending classes while you are pregnant, you give yourself the chance to meet other people who can relate to what you are going through. Resources and information can be shared, and lifelong friendships can be made. You also enjoy cyber relationships through online forums, where you and other expectant mothers can engage in discussions and share resources.

Take the time to share your attachment pregnancy experience with someone who understands exactly what you're experiencing.

## Your Coworkers

Many pregnant women spend a significant amount of time with coworkers, at least a few days a week. On an intellectual level, it may seem as though you have no control over who your coworkers are and how you have to interact with them, but it is important to realize that, like it or not, your coworkers influence your daily life and can either help contribute to your healthy attachment pregnancy or add to your stress level.

Yes, there may be coworkers in your life who gossip, complain, and emanate negativity. While you cannot control these people or avoid them completely, you can control how you let them affect you and your baby. Choose not to emotionally engage with anyone who isn't supportive of a peaceful lifestyle and pregnancy, and try to become aware of any coworkers who create drama or negative energy. Once you are consciously aware of who these people are and how you are affected by their behavior, take steps to change your mind about how you see them.

### Change Your Mind

How can you change your mind about how you view your coworkers? Well, changing your mind about how you feel about someone is not really as hard as you think. The first step is to begin to see how you are a participant in the actions that make you feel unhappy and stressed. Do you choose to participate in gossip? Do you choose to take things your coworkers say personally? Do you let things like reports and deadlines weigh down your heart, instead of allowing yourself to focus on what is really important in your life? Have you tried seeing your coworkers through your heart space?

Have you placed the priorities of your life in the right order for an attachment pregnancy?

## Look at Your Priorities

When your priorities are out of order, it is easy to let your relationships with your coworkers have an artificially inflated importance. For many people, once you really look at your life, priorities will often (though not always) break down something like this:

- Your relationship to yourself, your spirit, and/or your connection to your source
- Your relationship to your baby
- Your relationship to your family and partner
- Your relationship to your friends
- Your relationship to those things that nourish you and sustain your soul
- Finally, your relationship to your job and relationships with coworkers

If you are experiencing an imbalance, your ability to fully bond with your baby is in jeopardy, and it's time to make a change.

## Minimize Contact

Your next option is to minimize contact with coworkers who cause you to feel stressed, and in turn stress your baby. When negative situations with these individuals occur, remember that you have the power to choose how you react. You can observe their behavior consciously and choose not to plug in. There is no better time than when you are in these situations to practice Conscious Attachment. Talking with, or reacting to, these people only multiplies the negativity. When conversation starts to descend from real work-related information into gossip or blame, remove yourself. Practice Conscious Attachment. Focus on your heart space. Use your bond with your baby to help you navigate these difficult situations. Once the negative coworkers realize that you won't plug in, they are less likely to try and engage you into their future dramas. Dr. Wayne Dyer often says, "When you change the way you look at things, the things you look at change." Begin a work atmosphere renovation. You might even place a sign near your desk that says, "Baby attachment zone—no negativity!"

Everything and everyone around you affects your baby's development and the person she will become. By choosing to spend time with your positive coworkers and/or choosing to view your negative coworkers in a different light, you choose to have a less stressful workplace and a healthier attachment pregnancy for you and your baby.

## Your Spiritual Support

Pregnancy is a time when you begin to make observations about who you are, why you are here, and how you want to raise your child. During this time you may decide to seek out or deepen your spiritual connection and spiritual support. As your bond with your baby deepens, it becomes natural to think about how you want to support and raise your baby in a spiritual sense.

Spiritual support means something different to everyone. Simply put, your spiritual support can be anyone or anything that helps you feel connected to your source, something or someone who gives you purpose. Your support can be a traditional church and clergy, or it can be an activity that is very private and just between you and your source. Whatever means of spiritual support you seek, it should provide you with comfort and peace, not become a source of guilt and shame. You may want church attendance to be a tradition/ritual that you instill in your child. Being a part of a congregation of like-minded people may offer you support and comfort. However, you may find a private relationship with your source feels more spiritual and connective to you. For example, some people use various forms of meditation, such as silent prayer, mindful breathing, or ritual, as their connection to their source.

No matter how you choose to connect to your source, what is vital to attachment pregnancy is that it feels good to you. You want to find and connect to whatever it is that provides you with joy, love, and connection. There are really only two ways of functioning in the world: acting out of fear or acting out of love. Deepening the connection to your source during pregnancy helps you to act from a loving space, which deepens your attachment to your baby. When you are acting out of love, you are at peace and the womb is also a peaceful place. This is the best environment for attachment pregnancy.

> **"Ask and it shall be given to you, seek and ye shall find, knock and it shall be opened to you."**
> ~Matthew 7:7, the Holy Bible: King James Version

## Prayer and Meditation

Science has recognized the real power of prayer and meditation in positively influencing the body and mind. There are benefits no matter what theological belief system the prayer stems from. Taking moments to become quiet and connect to your source offers amazing benefits for the attachment pregnancy. Prayer and meditation provide you with the ability to be in a quiet and open state where you can communicate directly to your source and your baby. You also have the opportunity to seek spiritual guidance for important decisions regarding you and your baby. While the meditation practices referred to in Chapter 3 can be used without a specific desire to connect to source, the fact is that the state of meditation and prayer creates a state of mind that helps you communicate with your source regardless of your intention. According to recent research, the keys to successful prayer and meditation are as follows:

- You must believe in your connection to source when you pray or meditate
- Prayer is not about asking for something from your source; rather, it is about surrendering the situation to your source to allow the highest good to manifest
- Prayer connects you to the loving influence of your source
- Nondirected prayer (praying for whatever is in the highest good of all versus a direct prayer, which is asking for something specific) has the most potential for change and love
- Prayer is limitless, timeless, and always available

During pregnancy, you are teaching your baby about how to be in relationships for the rest of her life. When you choose to have relationships grounded in trust, security, and love, you are teaching your child that the world is a safe and secure place. This is the foundation of attachment, offering a safe haven and secure bond for your baby to begin her life.

> "May your Spirit, which is within me, so guide my thoughts, my feelings, and my perceptions of all things that I might grow into a happier, more peaceful, more loving human being. Illumine my mind, illumine my life. Amen."
> ~Marianne Williamson, Author of *Illuminata: A Return to Prayer*

# CHAPTER SUMMARY

Your conscious awareness of your relationships during the first trimester and how you choose to engage or disengage will ultimately impact your attachment pregnancy. When your relationships are a source of positive support, it supports an optimal state of mind for attachment pregnancy. Remember:

- You can consciously choose to create a deeper bond with the people in your life who positively impact you, or you can choose to limit those relationships that have a negative impact. This helps your baby feel protected, safe, and secure.

- Your perceptions of your relationships become your child's perceptions. The current health of your family is the basis for the health of the family you are creating.

- Forgiveness is about freeing yourself from the bondage of negative emotions you feel toward someone; forgiveness is not about absolution of guilt. Choosing to forgive does not change the past; rather, it frees you from the negative emotions of past events.

- You have no control over other people's actions. Wishing things would change is wasted energy. You can only change your response to them and how you see the situation.

- Your ability to bond with others and have a close circle of friends will help you to securely bond with your baby. When you focus on friendships where you can engage in a high level of trust, sharing, and hope, you create a higher level of personal satisfaction and security in your life. These qualities enhance the motherbaby bond.

- When your personal priorities are out of order, it is easy to let less-significant relationships have an artificially inflated importance. If you are experiencing this imbalance, your ability to fully bond with your baby is in jeopardy.

- Whatever means of spiritual support you seek, it should provide you with comfort and peace and feel good to you, not become a source of guilt and shame.

- Deepening the connection to your source during pregnancy helps you to act from a loving space, which deepens your attachment to your baby.

- Prayer and meditation provide you with the ability to be in a quiet and open state where you can communicate directly to your source and your baby.

- Prayer is not about asking for something from your source; rather, it is about surrendering the situation to your source to allow the highest good to manifest.

# PART 3

# Nourishing: The Second Trimester of Pregnancy

## BO**N**D
### N stands for Nourishing

"When you recover or discover something
that nourishes your soul and brings
you joy, care enough about yourself to
make room for it in your life."

~Dr. Jean Shinoda Bolen,
Author, Jungian Therapist, and Women's Activist

An attachment pregnancy is about understanding and honoring the motherbaby bond. As your pregnancy progresses, you begin to realize that the more you care for and nourish yourself, the more your baby is nourished. This early relationship between you and your child will be the first guiding map for your baby to navigate her emotional world. The attachment you develop with your baby, as well as the relationship you have with your partner during pregnancy, provide the first stepping stones for your baby's capacity to trust and nourish herself throughout her life. Your ability to manage stress, become mindful of your emotions, and practice self-care by engaging in healthy habits like napping and eating well contributes to your baby's healthy development on many levels. Loving yourself through self-nurturing equates to loving your baby in an attachment pregnancy. Throughout this part, you'll learn how to nourish yourself, your relationship with your partner, and your baby through your attachment pregnancy.

# CHAPTER 10

# Nourishing Yourself and Your Baby

> "Why are we here? We exist not to pursue happiness, which is fleeting, or outer accomplishment, which can always be bettered. We are here to nourish the self."
>
> ~Deepak Chopra, MD, Global Leader and
> Pioneer in the Field of Mind/Body Medicine

The motherbaby bond is cultivated early in your pregnancy as you nourish your mind, body, and spirit. Your intentions, actions, and who and how you love play a vital role in your baby's development and the degree of attachment you and your baby feel in the second trimester. Your baby's sensory organs begin to develop, along with her awareness of the world that lies outside the womb. She begins to know you through your habits, routines, and emotions. She becomes more consciously attached to you with each passing day. During the second trimester, everything you experience in your world will form what your baby knows of the world. Your baby shares the flavors of food you taste, the sound of the music you listen to, and the feelings of love you have for her and others in your life. How will nourishing help you have a healthy and attached second trimester? You will find out in the next chapters.

## Why During Pregnancy?

When you choose a nourishing environment for yourself, it also enriches your baby's world. Even at this early stage, your baby is conscious and responding to love and attention, or the lack thereof. The second trimester is when you begin to feel not only an emotional connection but a physical connection to your baby; these first movements you feel in the womb are sometimes called *quickening*. This quickening is frequently the wake-up call that there really is a person connected and attached to you. For most it solidifies the primal attachment and protection instinct of the motherbaby bond. During this time period, your baby begins to respond to sounds, movement, voices, and your emotions by crying, smiling, and thumb-sucking. The miracle of the motherbaby bond unfolds and deepens during the second trimester, as your heart, mind, and body constantly communicate with your baby.

### Your Baby's Emotional Life

Every experience your baby has as a result of the motherbaby bond forms the foundation for all she perceives about the world. You love your baby and you want her to have a positive outlook on life, have healthy relationships, be loving and kind, and enjoy life. Pregnancy and the first years of your baby's life will be the most influential time when you can invest in who your child will become and what her world-view will be. Your baby's brain, though still very immature, is developing at astounding rates during the second trimester. At this point in your baby's life, her brain changes based on environmental factors that you are exposed to. Every thought you have and every emotion you feel is communicated directly to your baby, and every experience your child has in the womb changes the wiring of her brain. She begins to understand the world outside based on what your emotions communicate to her. The more you experience an emotion or situation, the more your brain is designed to expect that emotion or situation.

This prenatal period has the most impact on her emotional health, because your baby's emotional center in the brain, the limbic system, develops during this trimester. When you practice an attachment pregnancy and engage in positive emotions yourself, you consciously develop your child's brain to form a positive mental attitude. During the second trimester, the lobes of your baby's brain are developing and the brain wave activity is also increasing. During your pregnancy your baby's brain is in the delta brain wave mode. This mode is one of deep sleep and regeneration, and it is in this brain wave pattern that humans report experiencing the deepest connection to their source and the collective unconscious. This developmental period is one where your baby is in a constant state of feeling. You, as a mother, have a lot of creative power during this time to offer the deepest love and joy to your baby.

The delta brain phase connects your baby to her subconscious mind. This is the part of the mind that will form your baby's habits and core beliefs about the world and will rule her behavior and the majority of her thoughts for life. The subconscious always functions in the present tense, meaning that the subconscious mind cannot differentiate experiences in the past from experiences in the present. This means your baby's emotional experience during your pregnancy, as her subconscious mind is forming, will be the emotional story her mind tells her over and over again for the rest of her life. As a mother, you have the power to write this beginning chapter of her story, and to make it a tale of security, safety, and happiness.

As we discussed, the subconscious mind is formed based on emotional states, not intellectual thought. It is the mind of emotions and feeling. This means that, if your baby has a prenatal experience filled primarily with stress and anxiety, her brain will be set to expect anxiety and stress throughout her life. Alternatively, if she often experiences rushes of love and joy hormones, her mind will be set to anticipate love in her world.

## Prenatal Stress and Your Baby

The first part of your baby's brain to develop is the limbic system, which includes the amygdala and hippocampus, also known as the primitive brain regions. These parts of the brain activate our "gut reactions" and are necessary for human survival. The primitive brain processes memory, emotion, and reactions to stress. Chronic stress in a mother can alter the healthy development of these parts of the brain in her baby because the emotions your baby experiences during pregnancy begin the intricate wiring of her brain. This is how the human brain adapts itself for survival outside the womb; your baby is in constant preparation for the world she will encounter when she is born. Studies have shown that the degree of attachment and the level of stress in the prenatal environment impact your baby's brain size, her long-term risk of disease, her ability to reason later in life, and can even determine when she is born.

### The Hongerwinter Study

One of the most significant studies on stress and pregnancy was the Hongerwinter study. This study looked at the children born to the women who experienced the Dutch famine of 1944. During this time the Netherlands was occupied by the Nazis, and nearly 20,000 people died of starvation. Women who were pregnant during this period experienced terribly high levels of stress and starvation. Researchers were surprised to learn that not only were the babies born to these women smaller, but these children's offspring were also smaller. The babies' experiences in the womb actually changed the genetic expression of these babies, meaning that their physical and mental health was altered. Additionally, these children were more likely to experience schizophrenia, bipolar disorder, and other mental disorders directly related to the high levels of stress of their mother. During pregnancy, their brains became conditioned to expect the world to be a stressful and scary place.

This study's results have been replicated many times over in different cultures throughout our recent history. There is a definitive link between high levels of stress in pregnancy and alterations in the baby's brain chemistry and genetic expression. When mothers are highly stressed, their ability to bond with their baby is diminished, and this has real physical and genetic results that can last for generations. Studies have looked at babies born during China's Great Leap Forward, the Iraq War, and children in utero during the attacks on the United States on September 11, 2001. Each of these studies had similar results: When pregnant women experienced high stress levels, their babies were impacted. These studies showed a variety of effects that included, but were not limited to, premature birth, changes in brain chemistry and mental health, and increased risk of heart disease.

Babies are not shielded from their mother's stress; they take it as a cue for what their future has in store for them. Babies begin to prepare for that future while they are still in the womb. While it is unlikely that you will experience a stressor such as the terrible events mentioned, you still might be in a state of chronic stress due to today's high-paced, output-focused, high-demand society. When you are in a chronic state of stress, you are much less likely to engage in behaviors that are nourishing to yourself and your baby. Remember that you have already learned many ways to manage stress, such as meditation, smiling, yawning, and deep breathing, and practicing these activities will help you better nourish your attachment pregnancy.

It is important to pay attention to how you are feeling and how your body is reacting to life's stressors so that you can help your baby develop a healthy, strong brain that is wired with many positive neural connections. This early brain development is critical for setting the tone for all of your baby's future emotional experiences, and every emotional response to the world, including your baby's capacity to love, is directed by this primitive part of her brain.

## Love

The human capacity to love, both giving and receiving, is something that only develops from the time of conception through the toddler years. If humans do not experience a deep attachment and love from those caring for them during their formative years, the lifelong results can be detrimental. In fact, the most basic need for human babies, stronger even than the need for food, is the need to be loved. This need is in place from very early in pregnancy and is nurtured by the motherbaby bond. Some studies have shown that baby mammals, when forced to make a decision between food and love, will choose to receive love. In fact, in humans, the lack of love received as a baby and toddler is a known cause of Attachment Disorder. Love is vital to growth and the cornerstone for attachment. Creating healthy love connections for your child prenatally is easy: send her love! Ways to send your baby love include:

- Practice Conscious Attachment as often as possible
- Talk to your baby
- Sing to your baby
- Think loving thoughts about your baby while meditating
- Write love letters to your baby
- Read to your baby

Your love for your baby is limitless and always available and can be shared with your baby in a variety of ways for abundant reward.

"Love is the capacity to take care, to protect, to nourish. If you are not capable of generating that kind of energy toward yourself—if you are not capable of taking care of yourself, of nourishing yourself, of protecting yourself—it is very difficult to take care of another person . . . it's clear that to love oneself is the foundation of the love of other people. Love is a practice. Love is truly a practice."

~Thich Nhat Hanh, Zen Buddhist Monk

### Practice Conscious Attachment

Part of the reason that Conscious Attachment fosters an attachment pregnancy in the second trimester is that when you experience the emotion of love your brain releases oxytocin, the bonding or love hormone. Humans release this hormone at critical bonding moments including:

- falling in love
- experiencing loving touch
- experiencing orgasm
- giving birth
- breastfeeding
- connecting to and being present with those you love

Oxytocin excites the part of the brain that creates attachment. The flood of this hormone that you and your baby feel during the critical bonding moments affects the emotional center of the brain, and you and your baby experience the feeling of love. The more your baby experiences rushes of oxytocin from your loving thoughts during pregnancy, the more her brain becomes wired to expect, desire, and reciprocate love. This is how very early attachment occurs. Before your baby is born, you are creating attachments.

## Your Baby Communicates

Researchers have discovered that, when your baby experiences emotions, she communicates those emotions back to you via a series of complex hormonal reactions through the umbilical cord and placenta. The two of you share an emotional experience.

The more you send love to your baby, the more she sends love back to you. Alternatively, your baby also can feel your fears, anger, and anxieties. Don't let this worry you too much. In fact, allowing yourself to have a healthy array of emotions helps your child to create emotional intelligence (EQ). Babies should experience the full range of your emotions in pregnancy for optimal health. In fact, when babies experience short-term stress in the womb, they learn to become stress hardy. It is only when stress is chronic and unrelenting that it has a negative effect on your baby. Stress is normal, natural, and a healthy part of pregnancy. However, an attachment pregnancy thrives when stress is managed, short-lived, and not chronic.

The key to creating a healthy EQ in your baby is to allow yourself to fully experience your emotions, and then, if it is not an emotion that nourishes you and your baby, release it. To return your mind to a peaceful state after experiencing a stressful event, use the stress-relieving techniques discussed in Chapter 7.

## Fathers and Partners

Fathers and partners are not left out of the love equation. Your relationship with your primary partner during pregnancy has a significant impact on your baby. During the second trimester, your baby can hear and she begins to associate the voice of your partner with the emotions you experience when around him or her. Your child starts to have a relationship with her father (or your partner) well before she is born. So what does this mean about your relationship with your partner? It means there is no better time than now to develop a more loving, communicative, and deep relationship with the person who will be parenting with you. The next chapter will cover how to develop and strengthen your partner relationship.

## What's Up, Baby?

During the second trimester, your attachment pregnancy begins to feel more real, not only to you but also to those around you. As your belly begins to expand and there is visual evidence of your growing baby, you will also experience the first physical evidence of your baby when you begin to feel her movements. These tangible reminders of your baby make you feel even more emotionally connected to her. This increased bond helps you to remember how important it is to nourish yourself and your baby. During this trimester your baby's senses are maturing—tasting, smelling, hearing, touching. Your ability to communicate with your baby on these levels is heightened. This section highlights all of the remarkable ways your baby is developing during this trimester.

### Weeks Thirteen to Sixteen:

During the thirteenth to sixteenth weeks, lanugo, a fine hair, begins to develop on your baby's body and your baby's bones and muscle tissue begin to develop. By fifteen weeks, the development of the external genitals is complete. Though your baby's vision is limited, it is functional at this stage. Your baby's sense of touch also becomes more refined, and she can use her hands to interact with the things in her environment, including the umbilical cord, her mouth, or her twin brother or sister. Taste buds are developed by week fourteen, and it is believed that babies can taste at this stage. Your baby will gulp faster with sweet flavors in the amniotic fluid (from the foods you eat) and she'll swallow more slowly when there are bitter or sour flavors present. She is experiencing taste for the first time, and you are sharing the flavors of your foods with her. Your baby's sense of smell is functioning, and though your baby "smells" in a different way than she will when she is born, she experiences up to 120 different smell compounds. By week sixteen, reactive listening begins, before the ear has even completed its development. This means your baby reacts to sounds outside the womb. You can now share your love of music and read aloud to your baby, knowing that these actions strengthen your bond.

### Weeks Sixteen to Twenty:

During the sixteenth to twentieth weeks, your baby will grow to be about 9 inches long from head to foot. She will have eyelashes and eyebrows. You may feel quickening—the first movement of your baby inside you—around sixteen weeks. In addition, her sense of vision is developing and she is starting to have very basic eye movements. Her ability to hear is fully functional by eighteen weeks. Twins have been observed kissing and stroking one another at this stage.

### Weeks Twenty to Twenty-Four:

During this time period, your baby's finger- and footprints are developing. Her lungs begin to mature. Her ear structure is complete. The most important sound to your baby is the sound of your voice. Your baby responds to sounds outside the womb and reacts to those sounds.

### Weeks Twenty-Four to Twenty-Seven:

During these weeks, your baby will grow to be about 15 inches long from head to foot and will weigh about 2 pounds, 11 ounces. Her eyelids will begin to open. Her respiratory system has developed enough to allow for gas exchange, and her lungs are beginning to produce surfactant, a substance that will help her breathe when she is born. She begins to inhale and exhale the surrounding amniotic fluid to prepare for breathing at birth. Her sense of balance and position is complete. Her taste buds are refining, and her palate is expanding based on the flavors in the amniotic fluid, which change depending on your diet. This is also the age when your baby will start growing hair on her head. She will also begin to sleep and wake in regular patterns

By nourishing yourself through stress reduction and mindful attention to your emotions, you nourish your baby in so many ways. You are helping to develop your baby's EQ and encouraging your baby's brain to mature in a healthy way. An attachment pregnancy will prepare you to respond not only to your baby's needs in the future but also to your own needs, to be the best mother you can be.

# CHAPTER SUMMARY

Your ability to nourish yourself and your baby through your intentions, actions, and who and how you love are key factors in your baby's development and influence the degree of attachment you and your baby feel in the second trimester. Remember:

- Your baby is conscious and responding to love and attention in the womb. She has a profound emotional life before she is even born.

- This prenatal period has the most impact on her emotional health, because the emotional center of your baby's brain develops during this trimester.

- If your baby has a prenatal experience filled primarily with stress and anxiety, her brain will be set to expect anxiety and stress throughout her life. Alternatively, if she often experiences rushes of love and joy hormones, her mind will be set to anticipate love in her world.

- Choosing to practice an attachment pregnancy will help you consciously develop your child's brain to form a positive mental attitude by engaging in positive emotions yourself.

- When mothers are highly stressed, their ability to bond with their baby is diminished; this has real physical and genetic results that can last for generations.

- Pay attention to how you are feeling and how your body is reacting to life's stressors so you can help your baby develop a healthy, strong brain that is wired with many positive neural connections.

- The most basic need for your baby is the need to be loved.

- An attachment pregnancy thrives when stress is managed, short-lived, and not chronic. Some simple ways to manage stress during pregnancy include deep-breathing techniques, Conscious Attachment, smiling, and yawning.

- Your child starts to have a relationship with her father (or your partner) well before she is born. Choose to develop a more loving, communicative, and deep relationship with the person who will be parenting with you.

- During this trimester your baby's senses are maturing—tasting, smelling, hearing, touching. Your ability to communicate with your baby on these levels is heightened.

# CHAPTER 11

# Your Partner and Bonding

> "Even after all this time, the sun never says to the earth, 'You owe me.' Look what happens with a love like that: it lights the whole sky."
>
> ~Hafiz, Iranian Sufi Poet

Pregnancy will bring changes to your relationship that start now and will continue as your family grows and, in fact, the strength of your relationship with your partner and your perception of support from your partner has a great influence on the motherbaby bond. During this time, your feelings and your acceptance of your partner's feelings can strengthen your relationship or place a strain on it. After all, pregnancy is a time of rapid emotional and physical change for both you and your partner, and loving communication with your partner is crucial during this time to enhance attachment pregnancy. In this chapter, you will delve into your partner relationship and discover how the health of that relationship impacts the health of your baby. You will also learn how to identify with your partner's fears and communicate more effectively. Attachment pregnancy is not just about mother and baby attachment; it is about healthy attachment for the entire family.

*Note from the authors:* While we realize and honor the fact that not every pregnant woman has a partner, nor is every partner a man, we have chosen to use the terms father/partner/dad to describe the partner relationship. While some of the information in this chapter is specifically written for the father, much of it can be applied to other relationships, such as same-sex partners or single mothers who have a mother/sister/friend in a supportive role.

## Why During the Second Trimester?

During the second trimester, your baby can hear your voice and the voice of your partner in utero. Throughout this stage of your baby's development and moving forward, being consciously aware of your communication as a couple and expressing loving gratitude toward each other is far more important than you may think. Remember that your baby is a feeling person, and your baby feels your emotions. It only makes sense that your growing and developing baby is directly affected by the relationship you and your partner have with one another. In fact, your baby will recognize you both at birth because her relationship with both of you has been forming throughout your pregnancy.

Ultrasounds have shown babies in utero demonstrating a wide variety of emotional reactions to their fathers. These include smiling, grimacing, and showing body movements that indicate protection based on their mother's emotional reaction to her partner. Ultrasounds have also shown babies in the womb crying and reacting in fear after a simulated explosive fight between their mother and father. While it was once believed that these reactions were simply due to the babies' reflexes and that they had no relationship to their real emotional experiences, it is now known that babies have rich emotional lives in the womb and that they react physically and emotionally to their experiences based on the level of security and safety that they feel from their mothers' emotional reactions. If a mother is fearful or angry at her partner, the baby experiences that fear and begins over time to associate these feelings with the sound of the partner's voice. The same is true of a baby experiencing happiness and love when the mother is engaging in positive interactions with her partner.

Now, it is very normal in all partner relationships for there to be occasional disagreements, arguments, and general times of tension. In fact during pregnancy, conflicts can become more common due to added pressures. It's important for you to remember that, when you have a fight with your partner, your baby is an observer. After a conflict, it is important to minimize and resolve the emotional experience for your baby. This can be accomplished by calming yourself down, by practicing Conscious Attachment (see Chapter 4), and by communicating your love directly to your baby. In addition, when you and your partner are ready to resolve the conflict, you both should verbally acknowledge your baby's presence and your common goal for a healthy, attached family by saying something like, "Let's focus on our pregnancy and our baby and our desire to have a happy, healthy family." Then calmly address the issue and engage in loving interaction as much as possible.

Practicing loving and grateful communication during pregnancy only strengthens the motherbaby bond and your family by building a strong foundation for parenting after birth. The parental relationship is the first relationship most children observe and learn from and, in fact, most children learn to love by observing their parents' relationship. Children from families whose parents have a loving and nourishing relationship feel safer, more secure in their world, and attached to their parents, so make sure your relationship is one that you want your child modeling. How can you do this? Start by taking a look at your relationship and committing to making the changes necessary for a healthy family life.

## Look at Your Relationship

Does the relationship you have with your partner nourish you? Does your partner feel nourished in your relationship? The components of a nourishing relationship include both the giving and receiving of love, care, and positive communication. In much the same way that you cannot expect an abundant and plentiful harvest from an untended garden, you cannot expect your relationship to flourish when it isn't nourished and tended to with attention and love. When these aspects of a relationship are not protected, you can expect the relationship to wither.

During pregnancy you may feel pulled in a million different directions, and it is easy to misdirect your attention to things that seem urgent instead of the things that are most important. Things like work, household chores, returning calls and e-mails, and participating in social media are often the distractions that take time and attention away from your relationships. And, in fact, relationships often start down the road to neglect simply because life takes over and attentions become scattered. But it's worth putting the time into your relationship even if you're especially busy, because when pregnant women feel nourished and supported in their partnership, they are more likely to feel deep attachment to their baby. Ask yourself, what are your priorities? Is quality time with your partner more important than watching television? If your priorities are not with your partner, this could be an indication of being disconnected with yourself, your baby, your family, and your consciousness. It means you are in a state of unconsciousness regarding these relationships. Moving into consciousness in your partnership means becoming aware of your relationship habits—those actions you regularly do that, over time, either build your relationship or harm it. Practicing consciousness by being aware of these habits and making changes when necessary will strengthen your relationship. Even more importantly, it will strengthen your attachment pregnancy.

Your relationship with your partner is no longer exclusive between the two of you, as it now involves your baby. The relationship your baby has with her father during pregnancy is literally the relationship you have with him now. If you often harbor negative thoughts about your partner or find that you are feeling angry, or experience resentment or disappointment within your relationship, now is the time to address those feelings. Why? Because when mothers perceive a lack of support from their partner, it can diminish the attachment between mother and baby. The longer these issues are left unchecked, the more it affects your baby's future relationship with this person, your familial relationship, and the motherbaby bond. If changes are necessary, now is the time to make them. That said, physical or emotional abuse within a relationship should never be tolerated. If you are currently in an abusive relationship during pregnancy, please seek immediate assistance from local authorities or, if you're in the United States, by calling the National Domestic Violence Hotline at 800-799-SAFE.

## Strengthen Your Relationship with Gratitude

You want the best for your relationship, and of course you want the best for your family. This means finding ways to appreciate and feel gratitude for your partner and family. Gratitude for your partner is critical to a nourishing relationship. What is it you value about this person? What positive things does he bring to your relationship? In what ways does he care for you and your baby? Does he provide you with words of affirmation, quality time, receiving gifts, acts of service, and physical touch? These are the five languages of love that Dr. Gary Chapman addresses in his book, *The 5 Love Languages,* an excellent resource to help identify the ways couples can show love for one another. His book is based on the idea that everyone has a love language, which is the way a person communicates love. Dr. Chapman states that often partners speak different love languages and, in fact, are drawn to people who speak a love language other than their own.

Are you aware of your partner's love language? Do you express gratitude for the ways he shows he loves you and your baby? Even more critical, do you take time to feel gratitude for his acts of love? Begin today. Experience gratitude and love for your partner. Find at least one way your partner expresses his love and sit for a few minutes in gratitude for this act of love. Even better, tell your partner that you notice what he does for you and express your gratitude for these things to him, no matter how small. When you embrace the concept of gratitude in your partner relationship, you are more likely to feel closer to him. This closeness will help you feel more connected to him and want to identify with his feelings during pregnancy. In the next section, you will learn about the most common concerns partners have during pregnancy.

> "Encouragement requires empathy and seeing the world from your spouse's perspective. We must first learn what is important to our spouse. Only then can we give encouragement. With verbal encouragement, we are trying to communicate, 'I know. I care. I am with you. How can I help?' We are trying to show that we believe in him and in his abilities. We are giving credit and praise."
>
> ~Dr. Gary Chapman, Marriage and Family Life Expert

## Your Partner's Experience of Pregnancy

*Couvade* is a French term that means "phantom pregnancy" or "sympathy pregnancy." This syndrome occurs when men experience some of the symptoms of the mother's pregnancy, including backaches, weight gain, cramping, nausea, and sensations that feel like contractions. Some men even experience prenatal and postpartum depression. In a very real way, many fathers are just as "pregnant" as the mother is. However, the father's experience of the pregnancy is uniquely different.

Mothers often express feelings of concern that the father does not share her same level of connection to the baby during pregnancy. This is normal and due mainly to the different ways that female and male brains are wired and the different hormones their bodies produce. The female brain is designed to nurture, nourish, protect, and love her baby from the moment of conception. The hormones of pregnancy, such as oxytocin, prolactin, and estrogen are responsible for the increased feelings of nurturing, as well as the heightened emotions of the mother. The male brain is designed to care for his mate, provide protection, and develop a bond to his child once the baby is born.

It's very important for you to understand that this is normal for fathers. In fact, the hormones that create the bond between a father and his baby—oxytocin and vasopressin, respectively known as the bonding and monogamy hormones—are released at their highest levels when he is present at labor and birth, when he holds his baby and participates in caretaking activities, and when he is near the breastfeeding mother. Men are designed to do the most bonding with babies after birth, not before, though many dads feel a very close bond to their child during pregnancy. The closer a partner is physically to the mother during pregnancy, the more likely it is that the hormones that promote bonding will be elevated in him as well. You should not be alarmed if dad is not quite as excited as you are about picking out the crib or the color of the nursery; it does not mean he doesn't love you or the baby.

The good news is that the involvement in pregnancy, childbirth, and parenting for today's dads has changed significantly from the previous generation. Fathers are more emotionally and physically involved in their children's lives than ever before and are an integral part of attachment pregnancy. More than 90 percent of today's American fathers are present at birth, and fathers are more likely than ever to attend prenatal visits, go to childbirth classes, be active in selecting child care, or even be the primary caregiver at home when the baby arrives. However, this does not mean that their fears have disappeared. When you can understand and perhaps even identify with some of the fears that your partner has, it is easier to understand your partner's behaviors and reactions during pregnancy. Understanding breeds compassion and makes relationships that much easier. Common concerns of expectant fathers are:

## Your Health

Your body is changing, your moods are changing, and your healthcare needs are changing. Your partner is adjusting to who you are now. Dads report that the health of their partner is one of their primary concerns during pregnancy. Like you, your partner has had a lifetime of media influences depicting the inaccurate message that pregnancy is dangerous and birth even more so. He may harbor fear about your safety during pregnancy, labor, and birth.

## Financial Stability

Your family's financial needs have changed. This can place a strain on any relationship. Not only are there additional healthcare expenses associated with pregnancy and birth, there are additional costs to consider, including, but not limited to:

- baby gear
- the possibility of new housing needs
- the potential need for a larger family vehicle
- missed time at work

Of course, these are all in addition to the enormous cost of raising a child. The U.S. government currently estimates the cost to raise a child through age eighteen is around $400,000, depending on your income bracket—and this doesn't include the cost of college. Dads can become overwhelmed quickly because of their desire to provide for their family.

## His Ability to Father/Parent

During this time period, dads begin to think about what kind of father they want to be. They begin to consider their relationship with their own fathers, how they want to be like them, and how they want to be different. Just like you, and every other parent that has come before you, your partner may worry that he does not have what it takes. Discussing the fear of becoming a parent and the goals that both have for parenting is one way to address this common fear.

## Your Sex Life

Pregnancy changes your sex life. Period. Even though sex in pregnancy is generally regarded as normal, safe, and healthy, there are emotional and physical concerns for both partners. You may feel too tired, have a decreased sex drive, or be too uncomfortable to want to engage in sex. You may want to have sex, but dad may be fearful. He may have concerns about hurting the baby or hurting you. He may have an unrealistic idea of what the baby is exposed to during sex. You might be surprised to know that many dads have an unfounded fear that their penis will somehow come into contact with the baby and potentially cause harm.

Taking a childbirth class together can help you both understand the anatomy of pregnancy and process of birth, as well as reduce fears around engaging in intercourse. Sometimes couples find that it takes creativity and a willingness to try many different positions and intimacy options before they find what works best in pregnancy. In addition, you can comfort your partner with the knowledge that the hormone that is released during lovemaking is oxytocin, the love and bonding hormone. This hormone ensures that your baby is not stressed by intercourse; in fact, she receives benefits from the oxytocin that is flowing, so go ahead. Get your groove on! If you are worried about some aspect of sex during pregnancy, talk to your healthcare provider.

## Change in Your Relationship Rituals

Friday night date night, coffee at Starbucks, waterskiing at the lake together, sharing a glass of wine. These routines have changed, and dad may now be missing his connection to you. It's normal for both of you to miss aspects of your relationship that must be temporarily put on hold. Fathers may feel even more isolated because they don't have the social perks of pregnancy. The world loves pregnant women, but your partner does not have the physical proof of being an expectant dad. No one is rubbing his belly or asking if he is having a boy or girl. It's no wonder that dads often feel a little left out.

## Additional Responsibilities

In addition to your family's financial responsibilities increasing, there are many other responsibilities that will primarily become your partner's, including the ever-expanding honey-do list. There are simply tasks that a pregnant mom should no longer do, like cleaning a cat litter box (risk of toxoplasmosis), heavy lifting (risk of ligament injury), and painting the nursery (toxic fumes). Dads often have to work harder at their jobs because they are worried about finances, and they have even less time to relax during their off time. Now, not only does he have additional responsibilities during his time off, he will have even less time for the hobbies he loves. In fact, some pastimes may be eliminated altogether due to new priorities. For example, some dads may have enjoyed motorcycle riding. This may no longer be an activity that he will participate in after the baby arrives, due to a change in priorities like safety issues, available time, and cost.

Not being able to participate in activities that previously brought joy is something the two of you will want to talk about. Often new parents go through a stage of grief as they mourn the loss of their old lives. Letting go of who you both were as childless individuals can be a process. Take time to talk about ways you both can carve time into your new lives for things you can do and enjoy. Babies do change your life. While it's true that there will be a need to let go of many things, there are wonderful new things to come that can only be experienced as a parent, like the first time you both will hold your warm, snuggly baby against you or hear your child's laughter.

Now that you have some insight into the most common partner fears, it is time to start communicating about them. The best way to do this is to communicate in Conscious Agreement.

## Using Conscious Agreement for Communication

Conscious awareness of the communication style you and your partner use to talk with one another is important to nourishing yourself, your partner, and your baby. You need to talk about your worries with one another, which means being vulnerable. This can feel very uncomfortable. However, in a truly nurturing relationship, true communication is of utmost importance. If you choose not to talk honestly with one another about your feelings and concerns, you build a wall that separates you and hinders a nourishing relationship. If you create walls during pregnancy, it will be even more difficult to break down the barriers when the baby is born. The very nature of a wall means that there are two sides with a barrier in between. There is a "your" side and a "my" side, and no "our" side. Removing walls allows for "we" instead of "me." The most successful parenting involves embracing the "we" concept, as opposed to the "me" concept. Attachment pregnancy is a "we" concept all around. To ensure that your pregnancy makes use of "we," use Conscious Agreement when talking to your partner. Remember, using Conscious Agreement during communication involves being honest, truthful, and speaking from your heart. When you are using Conscious Agreement, you are speaking from your heart and not your ego. The ego just wants to be right, whereas the heart wants to be understood and loved. How can you use Conscious Agreement when communicating with your partner? Try the H.A.L.T. technique!

## H.A.L.T.

When entering into important discussions, first check in with yourself. There is a self-care technique called H.A.L.T. that can help you identify when to "halt" or stop conversations or important interactions. H.A.L.T. stands for being:

- Hungry
- Angry
- Lonely
- Tired

Important decisions and discussions should never be made when you are feeling hungry, angry, lonely, or tired, because when you are experiencing one of these states, you are more likely to say things you don't mean or that are intended to cause harm. Communicating with your partner when one or both of you is in a state of H.A.L.T. can lead to harmful and hurtful outcomes, because your body and mind are in disconnect. Remember your baby is present during all of your communications, and you are also likely to be out of touch with your baby's needs when you are in H.A.L.T.

During these times, rather than engaging your partner in conversation, you should "halt" communication and take care of your basic needs. Take a nap, eat a snack, or practice the techniques to release stress in Chapter 7. By practicing the H.A.L.T. technique, you can identify when you need to put off important and meaningful conversations.

## How to Communicate in Conscious Agreement

How you communicate with your partner can set the stage for a healthy and connected partner relationship. Learning strategies to better communicate can only improve your attachment pregnancy. Here are some tips to use when trying to communicate in Conscious Agreement with your partner. Remember, your baby is observing your interaction. Ask yourself if your communication with your partner is positively contributing to an attachment pregnancy. The relationship you have with your partner is affecting the relationship your baby will have with your partner, and the health of your family unit.

### Use "I" Not "You"

You want to speak in terms of "I" not "you." For example, "I feel very lonely when you play golf on the weekends and we have so little time together" versus "You make me feel like you don't care about me when you play golf on the weekends." The first sentence identifies only your feelings. It is not accusatory. It does not put your partner immediately on the defensive.

### Take Responsibility

You are responsible at all times for what you say and how you act, regardless of how others choose to engage and communicate. The old adage is true; two wrongs don't make a right. Even if you feel wounded or hurt during a conversation with your partner, it is important to not try and one-up him by saying harmful things back. As soon as you behave in this manner, you have moved out of Conscious Agreement and moved further from the relationship that you want to have. You have also disconnected from an attachment pregnancy.

### Stay in the Present

When communicating, talk about the specific issue you want to address. Do not resort to bringing up the past or discussing "hot button" topics that you know will upset you and your partner. Stay on task and be specific. Address issues as they arise, and when you can discuss them calmly. Don't let issues go unresolved, as this causes resentment between you and your partner and can make your baby feel unsecure.

### Observe Yourself

Observe yourself when you communicate with others. Are you communicating in a manner in which you would want to be communicated to? Are you yelling, name-calling, using force, blaming, swearing, threatening to leave your partner, or otherwise communicating in a destructive manner? Think about it: Would you want your child to observe and emulate this behavior? Remember, your baby *is* experiencing this behavior, even before she is born.

### Develop Your Listening Skills

Listening is just as much a part of communication as sharing is. True listening means that you not only hear what your partner is saying, but you also reflect back what you have heard. This is called *reflective listening*. Reflective listening does not require you to solve the problem or agree with your partner's point of view, but it does let your partner feel validated and listened to, which is what everyone wants.

Here is an example of a couple who is not using reflective listening:

**Dad:** I wish that we could have sex more often. It seems like it has been weeks.

**Mom** (not using reflective listening skills): All you ever want to do is have sex. You don't understand how tired I am.

Instead, try the following . . .

**Dad:** I wish that we could have sex more often. It seems like it has been weeks.

**Mom** (using reflective listening skills): I understand that you want to be more intimate; so do I. Since I am so tired this time of night, how can we compromise so that both of us can have our needs met?

**Dad** (using reflective listening skills): Honey, I know you are really tired. How about we make a date for Saturday morning and just cuddle on the couch right now?

Using reflective listening skills can make a huge difference in all of your relationships. There are many books on reflective listening if you feel that this is a skill you wish to develop further.

As you move forward in your pregnancy, the relationship you have with your partner has a very real physical and emotional impact on you and your baby. Cultivating a healthy relationship now will lead to a happier you, a happier partner, a happier baby, and ultimately, an attached pregnancy.

# CHAPTER SUMMARY

Your baby experiences people outside the womb, specifically her father, based on the emotional reactions and relationship you have with them. By gaining a deeper understanding of your partner's concerns and challenges during pregnancy, and by developing supportive communication skills, you will enrich your relationship and attachment pregnancy. Remember:

- Loving communication with your partner is crucial during this time to enhance attachment pregnancy.

- Being consciously aware of your communication as a couple and expressing loving gratitude toward each other is important, because your developing baby is directly affected by the relationship you and your partner have with one another.

- Babies have a rich emotional life in the womb, and they react physically and emotionally to their experiences.

- When you have a fight with your partner, your baby is an observer.

- After a conflict, minimize and resolve the emotional experience for your baby by calming yourself down, practicing Conscious Attachment, and communicating love directly to your baby.

- When pregnant women feel nourished and supported in their partnership, they are more likely to feel deep attachment to their baby.

- The relationship your baby has with her father during pregnancy is literally the relationship you have with him now.

- The more physically close a partner is to the mother during pregnancy, the more likely these hormones that promote bonding will be elevated in him as well.

- The most common concerns a father has are regarding his partner's health, financial stability, his ability to father/parent, the couple's sex life, changes in relationship rituals, and additional responsibilities.

- The most successful parenting involves embracing the "we" concept, as opposed to the "me" concept.

- When you are hungry, angry, lonely, or tired (H.A.L.T.), you are more likely to say things you don't mean or that are intended to cause harm. You are also more likely to feel disconnected from your baby's needs.

- To communicate in Conscious Agreement, speak in terms of "I" not "you"; be responsible for what you say; stay in the present; observe yourself when you communicate with others; and develop your listening skills (reflective listening).

# CHAPTER 12

# Taking Care of Yourself and Your Baby

"Be good to yourself. You are a child of the universe, no less than the trees and stars. . . . In the noisy confusion of life, keep peace in your soul."

~Max Ehrmann, American Writer and Poet

The second trimester can be a time of renewed strength, increased energy, and a general sense of well-being. The body often (though not always) has adjusted to the various pregnancy hormones, and morning sickness often lessens or goes away completely. Your belly has grown large enough to make your pregnancy visible to others, but your baby is still small enough to allow for comfortable breathing, moving, and eating. This is the time to focus your mindful awareness on your pregnancy and your growing baby. It's the perfect time to completely nourish your mind, body, and spirit, knowing that you and your baby will receive direct benefits from this nourishment. In this chapter you will learn how napping isn't just a luxury, it is a pregnancy necessity. You will also discover how music can enhance your motherbaby bond. You will also learn how to identify and eliminate unhealthy habits to help nourish you and your baby.

## The Necessity of Napping (and Sleeping)

Western culture has moved away from embracing sleep, a necessary and precious act of self-care, because so much emphasis is now placed on getting things done. Now "doing" has become more important than "being." For some mothers-to-be, napping may seem like a luxury or a guilty pleasure, but do not be fooled; napping is actually necessary for attachment pregnancy, and it nourishes your body, your mind, and your baby. In fact, researchers at Harvard University and the University of York and have found that, without adequate sleep, your body is prone to memory loss, depression, lack of sex drive, low blood sugar, and reduced energy. Sleep is vital, and this is especially true during pregnancy.

### Get a Good Night's Sleep

The most rejuvenating type of sleep is the slow-wave sleep state of delta that you want to experience at night, not during daytime napping. When you achieve this sleep state, it allows the memory center in your brain (the hippocampus) to transfer memories to the thinking part of your brain (the neocortex). Slow-wave sleeping also allows your brain to reorganize so that it requires less overall energy to function, leaving you with more resources for other activities while awake.

For better nighttime sleep and to increase your slow-wave cycles, here are some tips from expert sleepers and scientists:

- *Warmth and heat help you drift off.* Take a warm bath or shower. Cozy up in front of the fireplace. Cuddle up with your partner and discuss the best parts of your day.

- *Eat low-to-medium glycemic foods (like coconut milk and raw carrots) shortly before bed.* For maximum effect, eat these foods no more than four hours before bed to help encourage slow-wave cycles for sleep. A cup of chamomile tea is another great sleep aid. Nuts and seeds are good choices for low-glycemic snacks.
- *Vigorous exercise in the late afternoon also encourages good nighttime sleep.* After work, join your partner or friends for a swim, which is an excellent exercise for pregnancy. Swimming reduces impact on the joints, increases the heart rate, supports the weight of the pregnant body, and helps your baby get lined up in the best position for her birth. Alternatively, you can take a brisk walk every night after dinner. Walk with your partner or friends; it's a great time to process the events of the day, share your dreams for parenting, and talk about things that really matter. If you are walking alone, it's a great time to practice Conscious Attachment.

A good night's sleep is certainly important—especially during an attachment pregnancy—but that doesn't mean that a good nap isn't important as well.

## Napping

You may think that daytime sleep, otherwise known as napping, isn't important, but it is, in fact, essential—especially during pregnancy. You see, the human body and mind function in cycles of energy called *biorhythms*, and you have high and low energy periods throughout the day. These biorhythms are designed to optimize your body's functions, including tasks like digesting, enhancing your immunity, regenerating your body's cells, and growing your baby. Biorhythms tell your body when to perform certain tasks based on the energy resources it has. Your body is designed to need a nap about eight hours after waking up in the morning. For most people this is in the midafternoon, between 2:00 P.M. and 4:00 P.M. During daytime sleep, you want to stay in a lighter sleep state for a simple, refreshing rest. Optimal nap times are fifteen to thirty minutes long. After the first thirty minutes of sleep, your mind moves from the alpha state into the delta state of deep sleep. If you nap too long, you can wake up feeling sleepy or sluggish instead of feeling deeply relaxed.

Rest in the form of napping helps the entire body relax. This allows you to wake up with more creativity, alertness, and ability to focus on your attachment pregnancy. If you are not accustomed to napping, you can start by simply paying attention to your body's cues. If you are feeling sleepy, rest. During rest and sleep cycles, the body is able to perform healing activity, release important rejuvenation hormones, and repair itself. When your body begins to signal you with signs of sleepiness (which is simply your body moving into a rest cycle), you might notice some of the following signs:

- Yawning
- Feelings of drowsiness
- Inability to concentrate
- Cravings for caffeine and sugar

It may be common for you to ignore these cues, and perhaps you have used crutches such as caffeine and sugar to keep going even when your body was telling you to rest. Next time you notice these cues, pay attention, and don't be afraid to close your eyes. If you are at work, set an alarm for fifteen to thirty minutes later, close your door, and turn off the lights. If you don't have an office, find a safe place to rest. Move into a restful position, put on an eye mask, and practice Conscious Attachment to achieve a relaxed state. If you have a sound machine or an MP3 player, you can play ambient sounds; you can even purchase music that is specifically designed to get you into a nap state more quickly. Soften your thoughts and relax into the wonderful world of napping. You are sure to wake feeling refreshed.

## Love Yourself and Your Baby

Sleep is essential and a necessary part of attachment pregnancy. You can love yourself and your baby by giving yourself permission to enjoy frequent napping and restful sleeping. When you are well rested, you are better able to nourish the relationships in your life, manage stress, and enjoy your attachment pregnancy. An additional benefit to becoming a prenatal napper is that you will be better at napping after your baby is born. Babies sleep throughout the day and have waking periods at night. If you become accustomed to napping before your baby is born, you will have an easier time napping when your baby naps once she is born. This skill will help you get a full eight hours of sleep over a twenty-four hour period. Studies show that babies who get plenty of naps sleep better at night. Guess what? Mommies do too!

## Sleep and Stress

In addition, you deal with stress better when you are well rested, and by now you know that stress management is a critical factor for an attachment pregnancy. If you feel guilty about napping at work, recognize that nourishing yourself will help keep your body and your pregnancy in a healthier state. It means you are less likely to need to go on bed rest, less likely to have preterm labor, and from the point of view of your workplace, you will be more efficient and productive after a nap. You can talk to your boss about taking a shorter lunch and using the rest of your lunchtime later in the day for a fifteen- to thirty-minute nap. Commit to daily naps to nourish yourself and your baby. Just as napping can become an enjoyable and stress-reducing part of your attachment pregnancy, music can be as well. Learn more about the stress-reducing and calming effects of music on your baby in the next section.

> **"A day without a nap is like a cupcake without frosting."**
> ~Terri Guillemets, Author

## In the Womb: Music and Your Baby

The sound of your heartbeat has been the background music playing for your baby since she was conceived. During the second trimester, you can also reduce your stress and enhance the motherbaby bond by playing music. Babies respond to music that is played during this time period because their hearing is developing and they are learning about their world based on their newly developing senses. Music that has a calming or happy mood has been shown to reduce stress in moms and babies; for example, babies respond to life-affirming music such as Braham's "Lullaby." Choosing music that mimics your heartbeat of approximately sixty beats per minute makes your baby feel comforted and secure. Interestingly, research shows that babies listening to rap, heavy metal, and even hip hop music show significant levels of stress, so try to avoid these as much as possible.

> **"I was born with music inside me. Music was one of my parts. Like my ribs, my kidneys, my liver, my heart. Like my blood. It was a force already within me when I arrived on the scene. It was a necessity for me—like food or water."**
> ~Ray Charles, American Blues Musician

Contrary to popular thought, when you play music for your baby, you should not place headphones on your belly. This is partly because this can make the music too loud for your baby's sensitive developing ears and partly because she should experience music through you. Part of your baby's musical experience is her exposure to the molecules of emotion that your brain is releasing in response to the music. If you play music loud enough for you to hear, your baby will be able to hear it as well, with the added benefit that she will experience your feelings relating to the music. If you are listening to music through headphones, your baby receives your positive molecules of emotion but she does not have the opportunity to experience the music itself. There is significant benefit to your baby being able to actually hear the music you listen to, so play the music you love out loud. Play music that makes you feel good, music that makes you want to dance. You can also bring music to your baby by trying the following:

- Pick some musical selections that you have a personal connection to. These selections should make you feel good when you listen to them. Try using this music to enhance your practice of Conscious Attachment. Enjoy knowing that you and your baby are sharing this experience.
- Learn a lullaby that you can sing to your baby. Sing this song to your baby every evening before you go to bed. Your baby will remember this song when she is born, and it can help her relax and sleep at night.
- Make up a fun or silly song with your partner that you both can sing to your baby throughout your pregnancy. Your laughter and positive molecules of emotion will deepen your connection with your baby and your partner. Your baby will also enjoy hearing the song once she is born.

The basic love of music and rhythm is innate in all humans. You can harness this feeling and use it to enhance your attachment pregnancy at any time. While incorporating music during pregnancy is easy and enjoyable, there are other actions you will need to take to truly nourish yourself and your baby that may in fact be challenging. It is time for you to take a look at some of your unsupportive habits in order to strengthen your motherbaby bond.

## Eliminating Unsupportive Habits

In pregnancy, your habits affect your baby's health, because everything you do during your pregnancy shapes your baby's brain development. You are also cultivating your baby's future habits through the habits that you practice during pregnancy and the early years of your child's life. At this point in your attachment pregnancy, you want to take the time to consider what habits you and your partner currently have that need to be changed, limited, or eliminated all together. Habits, those routine behaviors that you often engage in without thinking, that are not supportive to your attachment pregnancy are often a way to cover up feelings that you wish to suppress. Habits are part of your subconscious programming. They can be healthy or detrimental. Any action, such as overeating or smoking, that is not in alignment with loving yourself and your baby is a deterrent from your attachment pregnancy. By making healthy choices during pregnancy, you have the power to help your child grow to develop positive and healthy habits.

Identifying unhealthy habits and recognizing the underlying thoughts you have just prior to engaging in these habits is a great first step to begin eliminating them. Common unhealthy habits include, but are not limited to:

| Obvious unhealthy habits | Not-so-obvious unhealthy habits |
| --- | --- |
| Smoking tobacco or marijuana | Unhealthy diet |
| Overuse of caffeine | Overuse of electronics (such as cell phones, computers, video games, and TV) |
| Drinking alcohol | Sleep deprivation |
| Use of illegal or street drugs | Relationships with unsupportive or dangerous people |
| Habitual and unnecessary use of certain prescription and over-the-counter drugs | Routinely engaging in situations that cause chronic stress |
| Any risky behavior, unsafe sex, self-abuse, or mutilation | Working too much |
| Compulsive spending or shopping | Gossiping or participating in conversations that are negative, judgmental, or hurtful |

Often these behaviors are a way of making you feel "full," or emotionally satisfied. This sense of fullness is fleeting and not nourishing. The need for the feeling of fullness is what drives you toward these unhealthy behaviors. Your brain begins to connect the behaviors and the sense of feeling full in ways that make the behaviors habitual. Breaking habits is difficult, but it can be done. Many studies show that a mother's habits during pregnancy increase the likelihood of the baby developing similar habits as an adult. In fact, studies show that when pregnant mothers eat diets rich in sodium and sugar, their babies tend to grow up with a palate that craves these same foods. Whether you are aware of it or not, you are shaping your child's development and future habits. By making healthy choices during pregnancy, you have the power to help your child grow to develop positive and healthy habits.

## Breaking Bad Habits

The key to changing your habits is to first change the thoughts that led to your unhealthy habits in the first place. You must initially recognize that the behavior is not healthy or loving to yourself or your baby. Think about the emotion or feeling that is associated with a particular behavior, such as overeating. Does it initially make you feel good? Happy? Joyful? Numb? Next, think about the companion emotion. What do you feel after the behavior is over? Emptiness? Shame? Guilt? Sadness? Disgust? Regret? These negative emotions are a sign that you are not loving yourself or your baby fully. This ultimately means these habits are not beneficial to your family, your partner, and certainly not to an attachment pregnancy. Use the following activities to break your bad habits and replace them with habits that are healthy for you, your baby, and your attachment pregnancy.

---

### ACTIVITY: BREAK YOUR BAD HABITS

- Take a moment right now. Close your eyes and imagine how you feel after engaging in an unhealthy behavior. Imagine how your baby feels. Sit for a moment in the companion feeling that arises after the behavior is completed. Now take a breath, and imagine participating in a healthy activity that feels good to you and your baby, such as taking a walk outside. Connect with the feeling that this healthy behavior brings to you.

- Now think about which feeling would be more satisfactory as a long-term habit: the resulting emotion of your unhealthy behaviors or the feeling you get when you treat yourself and your baby lovingly.

- Take another breath. Now imagine yourself as a new you, a person who has new and healthier habits. Imagine how your baby feels growing inside a healthier and happier mother. Try to feel gratitude toward yourself, as if you have already made this change in your life. See yourself as already having made these changes in your daily habits. Imagine how your baby feels now that you have overcome this habit. Take pleasure in this sense of gratitude. You can silently repeat the affirmation *I am so happy and grateful that I now have* (insert your healthy behavior here) *as a healthy habit.*

- Repeat this activity daily as you are making your transformation. The practice of Conscious Attachment will help steer you toward healthier behaviors. The closer you feel to your baby, the more protective you feel and the less likely you are to engage in a behavior that could potentially harm her. The next step will be replacing your unhealthy habits with healthy habits.

- Once you have identified the behavior you wish to change, envision replacement activities that would create a feeling of fullness and contentedness in your life instead. These should be behaviors that are positive and healthy. What do you do that taps into your creativity and engages your soul and spirit? What do you do that makes you laugh? Do you like to write, cook, read, knit, do yoga, or exercise? The options are endless. These are all things that you can direct your energy toward to replace your unhealthy habits. Habits take about thirty days to form. You have around nine months or more to create healthier habits during pregnancy. You can choose to look at your pregnancy as not only the creation of a child and a family, but also the creation of a new you!

It takes time and effort to change habits. You must change your thoughts, your feelings, and your behavior consistently and repetitively to see real change. You need to replace old habits with new experiences. Don't get frustrated if you find yourself occasionally drifting off the path. It is normal and to be expected. What is most important is that when you find yourself off your new path, you correct the drift. This requires a renewed, daily commitment to your baby, your new path, and a strong resolve to stay the course. ●

> **"You're only a thought away from changing your life."**
> ~Dr. Wayne Dyer, from the Movie *The Shift*

### ACTIVITY: BUILD HEALTHY HABITS

Express gratitude to your baby! Take a few minutes right now to practice Conscious Attachment. Recognize how your baby is a catalyst for your positive growth. Thank your baby for helping you to make choices that are more aligned with who you want to be. Send love and gratitude to your baby. Stay in this loving space as long as you can. ●

> **"And the day came when the risk to remain tight in a bud was more painful than the risk it took to blossom."**
> ~Anais Nin, American Author

## Get Professional Support

It is always advisable to get professional support and assistance to help address unhealthy or dangerous habits. Talk to your healthcare provider for suggestions and/or see the recommendations in Chapter 2 for additional resources. Note that it is important to be honest with your healthcare provider about your lifestyle. Your doctor or midwife will only be able to recommend the right type of support and/or treatment for you if she knows the whole truth about your lifestyle. The thought of changing habits is not a comfortable one for most people, though some people find that changing unhealthy habits is easier when they know that their actions affect their baby.

You may feel a sense of shame or embarrassment associated with some of your unhealthy habits, and that is very normal. These feelings may deter you from openly communicating with your healthcare provider. Keep in mind that your healthcare provider has your and your baby's best health as her goal and wants to support you in your decision to improve your health. There are many kinds of support available for people who need to make lifestyle changes. Support groups, classes, religious or spiritual support, talk therapy, chiropractic and acupuncture care, nutritional counseling, and, in some cases, prescription medications are all options that can support you during your transition. By being honest with yourself, your partner, and your healthcare provider, you are giving your baby the very best version of you. Eliminating unhealthy habits can be difficult work and at times can diminish your energy. It is important during this phase to engage in activities that uplift and support you in your attachment pregnancy. This is part of nourishing yourself and your baby. Sometimes all it takes is slowing down to figure out your best course of action.

## Slow Down

It's easy to become overwhelmed with endless to-do lists and forget about the most essential preparation of all—nourishing yourself by slowing down and tuning in to the motherbaby bond. Many cultures around the world honor this period in pregnancy and encourage the motherbaby bond, so use their collective wisdom as a guide for your attachment pregnancy.

Traditional Japanese families believe that babies are influenced by the mother's thoughts, as well as by music. Pregnant Japanese women are encouraged to look at beautiful images, think positive thoughts, and listen to calming, beautiful music. In China, pregnant women are encouraged to avoid being critical of others, as it is believed any criticism will cause the pregnant mother's baby to take on these traits. Pregnancy is viewed as a time when a woman has happiness in her body. In Hawaiian tradition, babies are raised in the spirit of *Ohana*, or family bond. Babies and children are called *keiki*, meaning "seedling." Hawaiians wish to grow their children from the nourishing source of love.

## Experience a Blessingway

A wonderful way to honor your attachment pregnancy is to share in the tradition of a "blessingway." Sometimes combined with a baby shower, though very different, this ceremony originates from Native American Navajo practices to honor and bless the transition to motherhood.

The actual Navajo word for blessingway is *Hozho*, which has multiple meanings and encompasses all things good, beautiful, and harmonious. The blessingway ceremony honors the sacred rite of passage that a mother is going through. It can be a profound experience for all involved, and typically is a ceremony where only women are present. A traditional blessingway goes as follows:

- **Step 1:** The first step to the blessingway ritual is to organize a gathering of those who support and love you unconditionally. Often the ceremony begins with singing or storytelling and a lighting of candles. The first person lights a candle and says, for example, "I am Laurel, daughter of Jane, granddaughter of Louise, and mother of Trevor and Ryan." The next person lights a candle and shares her family story until the circle ends at the mother-to-be. Everyone uses her own candle to light one large candle in the center of the circle as the pregnant mother shares her story. These same candles can be lit again at a vigil during the mother's labor.
- **Step 2:** Next, the guests share something intimate with the group about their feelings for the mother and baby and their wishes for their future. Small and sacred gifts are given to the mother at this time. These gifts are typically handmade or of personal significance.

- **Step 3:** Next, the mother is given a footbath. Her feet are rubbed with blue cornmeal for purification and then soaked in a warm bowl of water that may contain essential oils and flower petals. During the footbath, she is given a hand and head massage.
- **Step 4:** After the footbath, there is time for storytelling. Personal and positive stories of courage regarding parenting, birth, and being a woman or mother are told. Sometimes a mother has her belly cast at this point, or has a henna painting done on her belly. Belly casting involves making a plaster mold of the belly and torso, which can be kept as a keepsake of the pregnancy. Henna art is an Indian tradition where the vegetable dye henna is painted in intricate patterns and symbols on the skin to celebrate a rite of passage.
- **Step 5:** The ceremony ends with sharing delicious homemade foods.

Some additional activities done at blessingways are:

- **Bead ceremony:** Guests bring a bead that symbolizes something they want to convey to the mother. The bead is given to the mother and a necklace is strung for her to wear during her labor as a reminder of her blessings.
- **Mother's wish book:** Guests have an opportunity to write something personal for the new mother and baby, as well as offer wishes for her journey into motherhood.
- **String ceremony:** A skein of yarn is placed in the center of the circle and a prayer or poem is read. The yarn is then looped around the mother's wrist and subsequently wrapped around the wrists of all of the guests. This symbolizes a deep connection between the mother, the baby, and all of the women present. The string is then cut and small sections are tied around each woman's wrist. The bracelets are worn until the baby is born.

The blessingway is a time when you can feel completely honored, loved, and celebrated. Many women are choosing to have blessingways instead of or as a part of a traditional baby shower. The celebration is a heartwarming way to step into motherhood.

> **"Take rest. A field that has rested gives bountiful crop."**
> ~Ovid, Roman Poet and Author

Taking care of yourself and your baby will be rewarding not only during pregnancy but also throughout your and your child's life. You are your baby's entire world. There is no other you. Your baby will learn to love and take care of herself by experiencing and observing you nourish yourself.

# CHAPTER SUMMARY

Your pregnancy is a perfect time to completely nourish your mind, body, and spirit, knowing that you and your baby will receive direct benefits from this nourishment. Remember:

- Sleep is vital, and this is especially true during pregnancy. Pay attention to your body's cues: if you are feeling sleepy, rest.

- Sleeping when you are tired allows you to wake up with more creativity, alertness, and ability to focus on your attachment pregnancy.

- Music that has a calming or happy mood has been shown to reduce stress in moms and babies.

- There is significant benefit to your baby being able to actually hear the music you listen to.

- Any action, such as overeating or smoking, that is not in alignment with loving yourself and your baby is a deterrent from your attachment pregnancy.

- Identifying unhealthy habits and recognizing the underlying thoughts you have just prior to engaging in these habits is a great first step to begin eliminating them.

- A mother's habits during pregnancy increase the likelihood of the baby developing similar habits as an adult.

- The key to changing your habits is to first change the thoughts that led to your unhealthy habits.

- You can choose to look at your pregnancy as not only the creation of a child and a family, but also the creation of a new you!

- It is always advisable to get professional support and assistance to help address unhealthy or dangerous habits.

- The blessingway is a ritual where you can feel completely honored, loved, and celebrated and can be an important part of nourishing yourself and your baby during pregnancy.

# PART 4

# Deciding: The Third Trimester of Pregnancy

## BON **D**
### D stands for Deciding

"Only the heart knows the true answer."

-DEEPAK CHOPRA, MD, Global Leader and
Pioneer in the Field of Mind/Body Medicine

You are your child's world. Every decision you make during pregnancy is changing your baby's world for better or for worse. There is no other time in the life of your child where your decisions have as much influence on the future health, happiness, and personality of your baby. In this part about "Deciding," you will learn how your wise nutrition choices in the third trimester direct the growth of your baby's brain and vital organs, how to safeguard your positive mental health, and how having parenting discussions with your partner now is essential for minimizing conflict throughout parenting. You will also discover how prenatal preparation for your ideal birth includes creating a birth vision board, communicating your desires, planning for pain-coping strategies, and selecting a supportive healthcare team and place of birth. Making good decisions about your labor and birth can help protect the motherbaby bond that you have created during your attachment pregnancy. The focus will then shift to taking time to imagine and plan for what life will be like when transitioning from an attachment pregnancy to attachment parenting.

# CHAPTER 13

# Decisions During Pregnancy

> **"Truly successful decision-making relies on a balance between deliberate and instinctive thinking."**
> ~Malcolm Gladwell, Journalist and Author of *The Tipping Point*

The third trimester is a time when you naturally move from imagination into reality. All of the dreams you have had about your baby are about to manifest into your new family. This is the time to make some concrete decisions about where you want to have your baby, what you want your labor and birth to be like, and how you and your partner want to practice early parenting in the first months of being a family. The decisions you make now can lay a strong foundation for family grounded in attachment, and your deep connection to your baby can help guide you to make the best intuitive and mindful decisions during this time.

## Nesting

As you move into your third trimester, you should know that it is normal to feel consumed by thoughts about preparing for your baby's arrival. Nesting is a primal instinct that most mothers experience as they prepare to welcome their babies. In the third trimester, you begin to withdraw from the business of the external world and start to prepare your "nest." As the hormones of nesting begin to take hold, you may find yourself in a state of reorganization and planning. It is easy to become overwhelmed with endless to-do lists and forget about the most essential preparation of all—slowing down and tuning in to the motherbaby bond. Paying attention to your baby's needs will help you make the best decisions possible. Use the following activity to take a look at what your baby really needs from you.

### ACTIVITY: MAKE YOUR NEST

You can do this activity alone or with your partner. It can be a great way to connect as parents, and plan for the arrival of your baby, by doing this activity together.

- Find a beautiful basket, bowl, or box that can symbolize the nest you are creating for your child.
- Reflect on all of the gifts you wish to give your child. Some examples might be security, love, happiness, attachment, and a sense of family. Find an item that represents each of these gifts; for example, a stone in the shape of a heart to symbolize love.
- Place these items in your nest. Make note that most of the time, the things you really want for your child do not cost money, but instead involve time spent with your child.
- Next, write a letter to your child sharing the meaning behind these gifts you want to give her and take a picture of your nest. This can be a wonderful keepsake.

Once your symbolic nest is completed, spend a few days reflecting on the actual nest you are creating for your baby. What does your real nest look like? Do your home and life reflect the qualities that you admire? What, if anything, do you need to change? Remember that attachment pregnancy is an opportunity to create the nest of your choice for your new family. ●

## What's Up, Baby?

As you make plans to welcome your newborn, your baby is getting ready for her exciting journey into a new world. Your baby begins establishing memory, experiencing rapid brain growth, and learning at astounding rates to help her transition to a new life in your arms. Your baby is highly tuned in to your world. Your attention to your baby's needs prepare her to greet her new world with trust, calmness, and a sense of security.

### Weeks Twenty-Eight to Thirty-Two:

During these weeks, your little one weighs approximately 3.5 pounds and will be about 16.5 inches long. She is sleeping and waking according to her own rhythms and cycles, regulating herself as her body continues to grow. She is experiencing rapid-eye-movement sleep, otherwise known as REM, which means she dreams while she sleeps. She already has a rich emotional life and her brain is rapidly connecting billions of neurons, shaping her idea of the world outside the womb. Her heart rate will respond by slowing down when you talk directly to her in a calm manner. She is deeply connected to your voice. Her milk teeth have developed below her gum line. Her eyes are capable of moving in their sockets, and she can follow the light from a flashlight shined on your belly. In fact, her eyes can even detect the differences between sunlight and artificial light, and her pupils dilate in response to changes in light. Her taste buds are maturing, and she can respond to flavors in the amniotic fluid by either gulping or grimacing. Your diet influences her palate, and eating a nutritious diet that is rich in flavor now can help your baby develop healthy eating patterns later on. Her lungs have developed to the point that she would have a great chance of survival even if she were born right now. The hair on her head is becoming thicker, as are her eyebrows and eyelashes.

Her body is also becoming more and more capable of functioning independently. Her bone marrow begins producing red blood cells, which transport nutrients and eliminate waste throughout her body. Her body is also beginning to store minerals like iron, phosphorus, and calcium, which will help her grow efficiently as a newborn. Your baby also begins to explore her own body by touching her toes, feeling her arms and hands, and grasping at her umbilical cord. This helps her become familiar with the sensation of touch. Her digestive tract is maturing, preparing for her first nourishing meals of colostrum (the newborn milk your breasts make). Toward the end of this period, her body will focus on creating fat stores and increasing the muscle mass in her tiny body.

### Weeks Thirty-Two to Thirty-Six:

Your baby is growing rapidly now, which means she is much more snug inside the uterus. You'll feel her movements intensely now, as there is not as much space for her to wiggle about. She has grown to approximately 5.5 pounds and can be up to 18.5 inches long. Your baby's genitalia are maturing; if you are having a boy, his testicles will begin their descent into the scrotum, and if you are having a girl, her clitoris is increasing in size. Your calcium intake will have a direct effect on the development of your baby's bones and teeth, so choose healthy sources of calcium for your diet like dark greens, hard cheeses, and fish with edible bones, such as sardines.

Your baby is learning how to digest by drinking amniotic fluid and urinating throughout the day. She begins to lay down fat stores in her body and gains about half a pound every week. Her body is beginning to regulate its own temperature. However, if she were born now, she would still need to be kept in constant skin-to-skin contact with you or stay in an incubator to keep her warm. She will open her eyes when she is awake and close her eyes when sleeping. Her immune system is being boosted by antibodies to prepare her for a new environment once she is born.

## Weeks Thirty-Six to Forty-Two:

Much of your baby's mature brain growth occurs in the last four weeks of pregnancy. This process allows her to breastfeed better, maintain her temperature, and interact with her environment. During these final weeks, babies often begin to make their way down into the pelvis head first, which is called *lightening* or *dropping*. Ideally, your baby will be positioned so that her back is rested against your belly and she is facing your backside. This is known as the *anterior position*, and it makes her journey down the birth canal easier when her birthday arrives. The fine hair that covered your baby's body, lanugo, is now disappearing and her skin is becoming smooth. Additionally, the white coating called *vernix* that protects your baby's skin from the watery environment is diminishing. She begins to store her first bowel movements, meconium, in her intestines. Her body has grown and prepared her for her destiny, to be your child. She is ready to be welcomed into your arms.

## Nutrition in the Third Trimester

As we've discussed throughout the book, one of the more important decisions in an attachment pregnancy is how you choose to nourish yourself and your baby. The food you eat actually signals certain developmental changes in your body and in your baby. There is fascinating new evidence that your placenta communicates with your brain to help direct the development of your baby. Your placenta produces serotonin, which helps aid in the development of your baby's pancreas, brain, and heart. If your diet is not rich in the foods that increase seratonin production, your baby's development can be hindered. An important essential amino acid for seratonin development is tryptophan, which should be plentiful in your diet during your attachment pregnancy. Some excellent sources of tryptophan are egg whites, chocolate, oats, dried dates, milk and yogurt, animal proteins, pumpkin seeds, and peanuts.

During the third trimester, your baby begins to develop her palate, or her taste for certain foods. The flavors of the foods you eat enter the amniotic fluid, which your baby can taste. What you eat affects your baby's future appetite. Research indicates that babies who are exposed to high levels of sugar, fat, and salt in the womb develop different reward centers in their brains. This means they become more likely as children—and later on as adults—to crave these unhealthy foods, which can increase their risk for obesity and other diseases. An unhealthy diet during pregnancy can also contribute to the development of diabetes and heart disease later in your child's life. In addition, there is evidence that eating foods that protect you from cancer-causing chemicals—including cruciferous vegetables (broccoli and cauliflower) and green tea—can also decrease your baby's risk of cancer later on. During your attachment pregnancy, you can create a healthy appetite and impact your baby's long-term health by consuming healthy and nutritious foods during the third trimester. Ultimately, your body is a reflection of your emotional health. When you love yourself by eating a healthful diet and paying attention to your baby's needs, your attachment pregnancy thrives.

## Eat the Colors of the Rainbow

It becomes very important to focus on eating a rainbow of foods during this trimester, not only to ensure that you are nourishing your body and your growing baby, but also to help your baby learn to love a wide variety of flavors and foods. You are your child's first teacher, even in utero. Teach her to love healthy foods and unique, nutritious flavors. It might be fun to try a new food every day. Try vegetables you have never tasted before. Sample fruits from around the world. Experiment with ethnic foods that you have never before tried. Most importantly, eat the healthy foods that your family normally loves to eat in abundance to help your child develop a taste for them. This will help you avoid the pitfall of having children who are picky eaters.

## Eat Fiber

Due to the fact that your expanding uterus and growing baby have taken up a great deal of space in your body, your digestive system literally has a lot of pressure on it. Ensuring that every meal has healthy fiber options can keep things moving! A diet high in fiber can prevent constipation. Examples of good fiber options include black beans, whole fruits and vegetables, nuts, and seeds. When you focus on eating healthy amounts of fiber, it helps your digestive system to function effectively. Healthy digestion means that your body absorbs more nutrients to help grow your baby.

## Focus on Essential Fatty Acids

Your baby's brain is growing by leaps and bounds during this trimester. In the last few weeks, her brain doubles in size and matures significantly, which means the neural connections in your baby's brain are occurring at incredibly fast rates. Her brain is primarily made of fat, and therefore needs essential fatty acids to grow correctly. How can you make sure she's getting what she needs? During the third trimester, focus on foods that are rich in essential fatty acids. Of particular significance is the omega-3 fatty acid DHA. An excellent source of DHA is wild-caught salmon. Studies show that moms who consumed more fish during pregnancy (at least four servings a week) had babies with higher cognitive developmental scores. Evening primrose oil (EPO) is another excellent source of essential fatty acids. EPO helps your body to produce prostaglandins, which are necessary for healthy digestion, fluid regulation, and healthy blood pressure.

Fish oil supplements can also be surprisingly beneficial for you during this trimester. They are rich with essential fatty acids that can not only help with your baby's brain growth but can also help benefit pregnancy. Studies have shown that ingesting fish oil can help reduce the risk of preterm labor and is associated with healthier weights in newborns.

Fish oil supplements can also help prevent postpartum mood and anxiety disorders, discussed in the following section. If you are not getting enough essential fatty acids in your diet, it can lead to mood imbalances and foggy thinking. Supplementing your diet with healthy fish oils can reduce this risk, especially if you do not eat enough fish in your everyday diet. Try taking a supplement every day that includes at least one gram of fish oil (though up to six grams during pregnancy is still considered safe). Some fish oils have added citrus to improve aftertaste. Check with your healthcare provider or registered dietician for the correct dosage.

## Perinatal Mood and Anxiety Disorders (PMAD)

While you may have heard of postpartum depression, very little media attention has been given to depression *during* pregnancy. Often perinatal mood and anxiety disorders (PMAD) begin during pregnancy, which is no surprise considering the fast-paced, high-stress lifestyle of today's society, coupled with the added demands of becoming a parent. These disorders can include depression and anxiety, obsessive-compulsive disorder, panic disorder, and bipolar disorder. In fact, there are estimates that between 15 and 23 percent of pregnant women suffer from depression. When the symptoms of PMAD during pregnancy are not recognized or treated, the risks for increased symptoms during the postpartum period are higher. Mood disorders can have a significant negative impact on the attachment pregnancy and also with motherbaby attachment in the postpartum period, so they should not go untreated. Making the decision to pay attention to your mental health and its impact on your attachment pregnancy is vital.

## What Are the Symptoms?

The symptoms of PMAD prenatally can sometimes be mistaken for common symptoms of pregnancy, such as insomnia, exhaustion, inability to focus (pregnancy brain), anxiety, worry, and fatigue. Additional symptoms that may indicate PMAD include a decrease in appetite, lack of joy, guilt, feelings of hopelessness, and an inability to feel refreshed after resting. If you experience any symptoms of PMAD, taking a proactive approach can help you navigate through this short period in your life safely and protect the motherbaby bond. Taking care of yourself prenatally and getting the treatment you need for PMAD can help reduce the risk of increased symptoms once your baby arrives.

## What Should You Do?

If you are experiencing any of these symptoms, understand that PMAD is a real illness, and like any other illness, treatment and support are important for recovery. Often, mothers can feel a sense of guilt or shame when they are experiencing the symptoms of PMAD and are hesitant to contact their healthcare provider or reach out to anyone. Understand that you are not alone; many women experience PMAD as a result of the hormones associated with pregnancy. PMAD does resolve with treatment.

There are many resources for women experiencing PMAD. As a first step, talk to your healthcare provider openly and honestly about how you are feeling. Specifically ask for a referral to a good therapist who can identify the best treatments for your symptoms. Don't assume your partner recognizes or understands the symptoms of PMAD. Partners need resources and information so they can be a part of your support team. Both you and your partner can find online support groups and resources. There are also excellent books and programs on the subject by Dr. Shoshana S. Bennett and Dr. Diana Lynn Barnes. Recognizing the signs of PMAD and taking the steps necessary to treat it if you are experiencing this challenge is an important way to maintain family health. Now let's discuss additional ways to keep your family healthy by planning ahead.

## Planning to Parent Together

The third trimester is the time to begin making plans for the arrival of your baby, and it's also the time to have the intimate and important discussions that matter to the long-term health of your family. As you begin these discussions with your partner, you might conjure up ideas about whom you think your child will be one day, how she will laugh, what she will do when she grows up. What are the two of you contributing to this unique little person inside of you? Remember that your (and your partner's) emotions help develop the emotional center in your baby's brain, the amygdala, and determine how she balances her emotions. When parents learn that their emotions help develop their baby's personality, it is common for them to begin to worry about times they have been stressed or angry during their pregnancy. Remind yourself instead to focus on your blessings at this time. Be in a state of gratitude as often as you can. Try to move from a state of mind of "it's hopeless" to "I am hopeful." Sit for a moment and begin to count your blessings. Focus on the many things that you have gratitude for in this moment. Having an attitude of gratitude can help keep you in a state of positive emotion. When having important discussions and making plans for your family's future, you want to start from a place of gratitude and positivity. These plans will form the foundation of your family. The more that you support one another as a team and have real discussions that matter, the more solid this foundation will be. Remember to use Conscious Agreement as a couple before entering into any discussion.

> "Whatever you are, whatever you do, your baby will get it. Anything you eat, any worries that are on your mind will be for him or her. Can you tell me that you cannot smile? Think of the baby, and smile for him, for her, for the future generations."
>
> ~Thich Nhat Hanh, from his book *Being Peace*

### ACTIVITY: PARENTING INTENTIONS

This is the time to begin to make decisions about issues that will impact you, your partner, and your baby. The more that you and your partner prepare for parenting prenatally, the more secure and stable your family bond will be. This activity guides you and your partner in a serious discussion about pivotal parenting issues so that you can come to Conscious Agreement before your baby is born. The following questions are meant to be a discussion guide, something that you do together. Use them as a starting point to begin planning your future family.

• How will we ensure that our family values focus around attachment and bonding for the family?

- How important is our family's nutrition and exercise? How will we support healthy nutrition and exercise as a family?
- Who will be primarily responsible for handling the finances of our family? What are our work plans for this pregnancy and after? How will our family manage any changes in finances?
- If we return to work after the baby is born, who will care for our child? Will we have the option of a friend or family member caring for the baby, or will we elect to use a day care center? How will that affect our attachment to our baby? Have we interviewed or visited any day care facilities? Are we in agreement on who will be the primary caregiver for our child?
- Is our current residence safe and appropriate for a new baby? If not, what are the plans for change? Do our finances support this change? What are all of our options for creating a safe, nurturing environment?
- What do we want our parenting style to look like? Will we practice attachment parenting? Will we co-sleep with our baby, or will our baby sleep in another room? What does "discipline" mean to each of us? Will one of us be taking on the majority of the caregiving, or will the responsibilities be divided equally? What are the roles and responsibilities of each parent (diapering, feeding, bathing, playing, etc.)?
- Have we decided upon our child's religious/spiritual upbringing? How big a role will religion/spirituality have in our family's life?
- What cultural traditions will our family observe?
- How will being a parent change our intimate/sex lives? Will we have a family bed? How will this change our sex life? Do we have a plan to stay intimate with one another?
- Which members of our extended family will have access to our child? How will we integrate our extended family into our lives? What level of influence do we want our extended family to have on our parenting styles, if any? What boundaries do we both agree will be healthy?

- When will we send our child to school? (Preschool can start as early as two years old.) Will we home-school? Will we send our child to private school? Do we have a plan for saving for our child's education?
- When our baby arrives, who will be responsible for the housework? What can be left undone? What aspects of housekeeping can we allow friends/family to help with? Can we hire a housekeeper?
- What are our plans for the healthcare of our child? Will our family seek out alternative or traditional healthcare? Have we considered things like immunizations, circumcision, breastfeeding, home birth or hospital birth, etc.?
- If we both cannot agree on a parenting decision, who has the final say? What will the process for decision-making look like? ●

As you move into your final trimester of pregnancy, your growing belly is a constant reminder of the fact that you are growing an actual person. Every decision you make has a direct and important affect on your child. Making mindful and loving decisions together in Conscious Agreement now will only serve to enhance the motherbaby bond, as well as the family bond.

# CHAPTER SUMMARY

The third trimester is when you should start to slow down enough that you can begin to examine your life and how it will impact your future family. You will begin the process of nesting, and that can lead you into a review of your self-care and how it affects your future family. Look at your nutrition and your mental health, and begin to have conversations with your partner about how you want to parent. Your deep connection to your baby can help guide you to make the best intuitive and mindful decisions during this time. Remember:

- Your attention to your baby's needs prepare her to greet her new world with trust, calmness, and a sense of security.

- The food you eat actually signals certain developmental changes in your body and your baby.

- You can create a healthy appetite and impact your baby's long-term health by consuming healthy and nutritious foods during the third trimester.

- During the third trimester, it is important to focus on foods rich in essential fatty acids to help with your baby's brain growth. They can also help with the prevention and management of mood and anxiety disorders during and after the pregnancy.

- Often perinatal mood and anxiety disorders (PMAD) begin during pregnancy. Taking care of yourself prenatally and getting the treatment you need for PMAD can help reduce the risk of increased symptoms once your baby arrives.

- Having an attitude of gratitude can help keep you in a state of positive emotion, which helps direct the development of your baby's brain in a healthy manner.

- Making decisions about issues that will impact you, your partner, and your baby prenatally will help stabilize not only the motherbaby bond but the family bond as well.

# CHAPTER 14

# The Bond and Birth

> "Birth is the sudden opening of a window, through which you look out upon a stupendous prospect. For what has happened? A miracle. You have exchanged nothing for the possibility of everything."
>
> ~William Macneile Dixon, Author and Prize-Winning Academic

Your labor and delivery is not just about you. It is also a very real experience for your baby, both physically and emotionally, and the experience of this sacred event offers opportunities to deepen the motherbaby bond after birth. Oxytocin, the love/bonding hormone, is at its highest level during the pushing phase of labor and in the hours after birth, the prime bonding time for you and your baby. While you have been bonding with your baby since conception, you want to honor and protect the first few hours after birth, as these are the first moments when you are face to face with your baby; this is your chance to bond with your baby on an entirely new level.

How can you prepare for labor and delivery? How can you protect these sacred bonding moments with your just-born baby? You have to do some legwork in advance. In this chapter, you'll learn how to create a birth vision board, pick your healthcare team, stay comfortable during labor, create a pain management plan, and much more that will keep you connected to your baby as your delivery date approaches.

## Keep It Natural

While sometimes medical intervention is necessary for your or your baby's health, when labor and birth are allowed to unfold normally and naturally your sense of empowerment and emotional health are increased, and you have the physical resources to care for and breastfeed your baby, which encourages a continuation of attachment pregnancy through the motherbaby bond. In addition, when your labor progresses naturally and normally, there is generally less risk of medical intervention. A medical intervention can include, but is not limited to, anything from a simple IV, to an epidural, to a cesarean birth. Intervention increases the risk of cesarean section and also potential birth trauma, which can delay early skin-to-skin contact and bonding. With normal and natural birth it is also less likely for your baby to need medical intervention, which can potentially cause her pain, exhaustion, sleepiness, and negatively impact bonding and breastfeeding. This is not to say that postpartum bonding cannot happen if medical intervention is needed or occurs, but it is not optimal for postpartum bonding.

## Create a Birth Vision Board

You can use the connection between you and your baby as well as your intuition at any time during pregnancy to help you make wise and healthy decisions. One way you can tap into this inner wisdom is through the creation of a vision board—a collage of images that you personally select to symbolize your wants and needs—that acts as a visual representation of your conscious aspirations and your subconscious desires. Sometimes people are not aware of what they really desire, and a vision board can help them "see" these things. During pregnancy, vision boards can help you tune in to the motherbaby bond and can be used as tools to help you shed light on the things that matter the most to you and your baby, and to clarify what is it that you really want. Typically what winds up on your vision board are the things that you feel drawn to in your life; these things are often part of your individual purpose. In a way, these boards are like a prayer or active meditation in that they can connect you to your source and illuminate your dreams, hopes, and wishes.

Using Conscious Agreement and Conscious Attachment (as described in the activity below), you (and your partner) can create a unique vision board that illustrates your innermost thoughts and can help you reveal the labor and birth that you dream of. A vision board can be your map toward a great birth experience for you and your baby, and it can even act as a great replacement for a traditional birth plan.

### ACTIVITY: USE CONSCIOUS AGREEMENT TO CREATE A BIRTH VISION BOARD

During pregnancy, your vision board will represent not only your wants and needs but also those of your baby. Before starting your vision board, honor the motherbaby bond by first practicing Conscious Attachment. This ensures that your vision board is a reflection of your attachment pregnancy.

- **Step One: Separate yourself from external influences (practice Conscious Attachment).** Go to a quiet place where you can be uninterrupted. Bring supplies like a poster board or a large sheet of paper, markers or crayons, magazines you love, pictures, scissors, glue, and anything else you might want to decorate your board with.
- **Step Two: Get quiet and pause.** Start by quieting your mind and beginning either meditation or prayer. Visualize yourself as a mother.

Visualize your baby. What does that bond look and feel like to you? How do you want this to be expressed in your labor and delivery? Try not to force ideas; just open up. As your intentions come to you, breathe them in. Feel them becoming a part of you with each breath. Stay in this quiet space for as long it feels comfortable to you.

- **Step Three: Listen in.** Pay attention to the visual images surrounding you. Begin by selecting the pictures or graphics that seem to resonate with your intentions. Choose words and images that you are drawn to and that make you feel good and portray your thoughts about your baby and your birth. For example, you might choose an image of a beach if that represents a feeling of peace for you. Next, arrange them on the paper into a shape or flow that appeals to you. Place a picture of yourself and/or an ultrasound of your baby in the center of your vision board so that the images surround you both, and the two of you are the center of all of these intentions. There may be blank areas on your vision board. This is okay. You may feel the need to come back in the future and add to or change your vision board. Leave yourself some space to be open to ideas that may still come to you.

- **Step Four: Decide and commit.** Once you have created your birth vision board, hang it up. Put it in a place where it is visible not only to you but also to those who are in your inner circle. Use it as a tool to discuss your hopes and your plans. Share it with your partner, as well as your doctor or midwife. Show it to your doula. Bring it to your birth. It's a piece of art that expresses your birth intentions.

You may wish to create a vision board surrounding anything in your life, your marriage, your parenting style, or your family. Date and save your vision boards; they will become unique historical journals of who you were when you created them. It is always fascinating to look back and see what your intentions were and how they manifested in your life. This is a great way to teach your children to tune into their hearts' desires as well. ●

## Labor and Delivery Options

Now that you have considered your wishes for your baby's birth with the vision board, it's time to make some decisions that will affect the future of your motherbaby bond and take a closer look at some of the options you will have during your labor and delivery. Keep in mind that these decisions are deeply personal and should be based on how you, your baby, and your partner feel, not the opinions of others. While having discussions with important people in your life might help you discover your innermost feelings, be careful to not be overly influenced by other people's opinions if they do not reflect your own desires. Before any final decision is made, go back and practice Conscious Attachment and Conscious Agreement, which are foundational for your attachment pregnancy.

The reality is that your attachment pregnancy will last approximately nine full months, and the motherbaby bond will last a lifetime. This may make the decisions concerning a typical twenty-four-hour labor seem comparatively less significant; however, your birth experience impacts you and your baby physically, emotionally, and spiritually. There is also evidence that the birth experience affects attachment as well. It is likely that you and your baby will have lasting effects from the birth experience for the rest of your lives. Therefore, thoughtful considerations of your labor and birth options regarding pain management, your healthcare providers, etc. are important for your long-term motherbaby bond.

### Perceptions of Pain

During attachment pregnancy, you should explore your feelings and options regarding labor preparation and pain management. If you are like most pregnant women, you have already spent some time thinking about how you will handle the pain of labor and birth. How you perceive pain and how you experience the birthing process will impact your ability to further bond with your baby.

This means that the more you prepare and create a support system for you and your baby, the better your opportunity is for bonding in the days and weeks following birth. Keep in mind that it is completely normal to have some fear about pain and the process of giving birth. Any time you are faced with the unknown, it is common to move into a fear response. But now is the time to reframe the way you think about pain in labor.

Pain is an unpleasant physical discomfort that can be a sensory or emotional experience. A woman in labor can be in pain and not experience suffering, which is the inability to emotionally cope with pain, fear, or the unknown because you feel that you are out of control. It is the *perception* of the experience that can cause suffering. Your ability to feel in control and supported can contribute to a more positive perception of your labor, regardless of the scenario. How you "see" the situation is what really matters. Consider these two scenarios:

- **Perception of suffering:** Your labor is progressing normally and you are moving from an active phase of labor to a transitional phase of labor. Your contractions are becoming longer, stronger, and closer together. You start to panic and fear for your safety. You withdraw from your support team and begin to wonder if you can trust anyone. You do not believe in your ability to give birth to this baby. You are terrified. You are suffering.
- **Perception of normal labor:** Your labor is progressing normally and you are moving from an active phase of labor to a transitional phase of labor. Your contractions are becoming longer, stronger, and closer together. Even though you are becoming increasingly uncomfortable physically, you know that you are in a safe place and that your body is functioning normally. You trust the people supporting you. You practice Conscious Attachment and connect to your baby. You lean on your partner for help. Even though you are experiencing a great deal of pain, you are not suffering.

It is the perception of what is happening that causes a woman in labor to interpret her pain as normal or as suffering. Through mindfulness and consciousness, you have the power to labor without suffering.

While labor can unfold in a variety of ways, and sometimes in unexpected ways, it is your memory of the birth that will impact the motherbaby bond. Your perception is key here, and your positive attitude and perception can help you tap into your intuition and allow you to make the best choices for you and your baby. Your memory of the birth experience will forever be with you and it can positively or negatively contribute to the motherbaby bond, largely depending on your perception. Your physical, emotional, and spiritual preparation for labor and birth will significantly contribute to your experience.

### What Is Labor Pain?

The pain that you feel in labor is different from any other type of pain you experience in your life. Unlike other pain that is a sign of illness or injury, labor pain is actually a sign that your body is working for you and your baby. The physical causes of labor pain include:

- movement of the baby
- stretching of your ligaments
- opening or dilation of your cervix
- pressure of your baby moving through the birth canal
- uterine muscle fatigue

Emotional factors that affect the perception of pain include but are not limited to:

- anxiety (which increases bodily tension)
- fear

- lack of support
- previous experiences with pain
- beliefs about your body and your ability to birth
- unexpected occurrences (such as medical interventions)
- a disconnect from your baby

Your environment also affects how you feel and deal with pain. When you have the support you need, the freedom to move around, the ability to use the comfort techniques of your choice, access to nourishment and hydration, and the ability to practice both Conscious Attachment and Conscious Agreement, you will find that your perception of pain is decreased.

### Subconscious Programming of Pain

Believe it or not, your mind has already formed an opinion about birth based on your subconscious programming. What you believe is based on the culture you grew up in and the media that you have been exposed to. Your belief systems regarding your body and birthing have a lot to do with how you will perceive pain during your labor. Close your eyes for a moment and visualize a woman in labor. Think about where she is and what she is doing. What comes to mind? Where did you get that image? Is this the way you *want* to give birth, or is it simply the way you think most women actually have a baby? The most common modern image of a woman laboring is one of her lying on her back and in terrible pain. It is not an accurate portrayal of the normal process of labor and birth. When you are in an environment of safety and security, your body is designed to help you and your baby cope with the sensations of labor and birth. Contractions are your body's way of bringing your baby into the world. Your body is working for you, not against you. Here are some myths and the realities about labor pain that will help you see what's real and what's your subconscious programming at work:

| Myth | Reality |
|------|---------|
| Labor pain is continuous. | Contractions are intermittent with rest in between. In a typical 24-hour labor, only 3 hours is actual contraction time. The majority of your labor is downtime. |
| Pain is unmanageable without medication. | There are many natural techniques and comfort measures that have been shown to decrease pain perceptions, improve relaxation, and shorten labor. |
| Labor is intense and fast from the very beginning. | Labor usually starts slowly and gradually intensifies. Your body has a chance to adjust and release comfort hormones to help with the pain. |
| Because women tend to vocalize or moan in labor it means they are in great pain. | Vocalization and moaning is a natural response during labor. It helps decrease the sensation of pain and softens the birth passage for the baby by relaxing the perineal muscles. |
| Pain is a sign that something is wrong. | Most sensation in labor is actually a sign that your body is working effectively. |

The emotional and physical commitment you make now to prepare for your labor and birth can contribute to a more positive perception of the experience. This can help reduce the risk of postpartum mood and anxiety disorder, increase motherbaby bonding, and ease the transition to life with a newborn for the entire family.

"We have a secret in our culture . . . and it's not that birth is painful. It's that women are strong."

~Laura Stavoe Harm, Writer

## Optimal Fetal Positioning

As we discussed in Chapter 12, pregnant women are encouraged to be as active as possible because of the wide array of benefits that exercise and movement offer. One additional benefit that we didn't discuss is the idea that movement can help get your baby lined up in the best possible position for your labor and birth. Optimal fetal positioning is a technique that was originally developed in the mid-1990s by midwife Jean Sutton and childbirth educator Pauline Scott. They discovered that maternal movement and positioning changes the way a baby positions herself in the pelvis and can improve the outcome of labor. The practice of optimal fetal positioning helps fine-tune your intuition as a mother and helps you be more aware of your baby. This process can also help you feel more connected to your baby due to the fact that you have to mindfully visualize your baby every day.

Toward the end of your pregnancy, your baby takes cues from nature and starts to settle into her birth position. There is very little room for her to move around in those last weeks and so she will find the most comfortable position. With the aid of gravity and the angle of your pelvis, most babies turn head-down. To visualize this optimal position, imagine your baby resting, head down, on the left side of your belly, with her back curled against your belly, facing your spine. This can cause your belly button to pop out, which is a good sign that your baby is in the correct position! This position, called an OA (occiput anterior) position, means that the back of your baby's head is facing your belly and allows the contours of your baby's head and shoulders to most easily fit through your pelvis during labor. This position promotes a shorter, easier, and less painful labor, which can enhance the postpartum motherbaby bond.

Unfortunately, today's lifestyle can include lots of sitting and resting in laid-back positions on comfy couches. When you spend a good deal of your time in these positions, it can change the way your baby rests in the womb. Due to the tilting of your pelvis in these laid-back positions, gravity pulls the heaviest parts of your baby (her back and head) toward your back instead of your belly. This is sometimes called the "sunny-side-up" position. Mothers whose babies lie in this position can experience painful back labor because they feel so much pressure on their back. This is called the OP (occiput posterior) position, which means that the back of your baby's head is facing your back.

In an optimal position, your baby's head is flexed and the average diameter of her head at your cervix is 9.4 centimeters, meaning you would only have to dilate to 9.4 centimeters to push her out. However, if your baby rests in the sunny-side-up position, the part of her head that is facing your cervix changes. In a posterior position, the diameter of her head facing the cervix is, on average, 11.5 centimeters. This means your cervix must dilate up to 2 centimeters more than if your baby was in an optimal position. In short, giving birth to a baby in a posterior position takes longer and is far more difficult.

### Help Your Baby Find an Optimal Position

You can begin to practice the positions that help your baby find her optimal position in the last six weeks of pregnancy if this is your first baby, or the last two to three weeks if you've already had a child. In general, you want to try and avoid positions that encourage your knees to be in a position higher than your hips (for example, sitting in most office chairs), and as we mentioned, you want to avoid lying back against comfy couch cushions, which enables your baby to rest against your spine and encourages a posterior position. Alternative positions you can try while relaxing include lying on your left side, using a birth ball, leaning over cushions, sitting cross-legged on the floor, or sitting backward on an armless chair and leaning forward. Place a rolled towel or wedge underneath your buttocks when you are in the car or at work, so that your knees are always lower than your pelvis. This creates the perfect angle for your baby to get in an optimal position.

Also, avoid practicing deep squats in yoga or exercise class until you are sure your baby is in an optimal, not posterior, position. Deep squats can engage your baby into the pelvis, and if your baby is posterior, she can get nestled deep into that position, which will make it harder for her to turn. Try to not cross your legs, as this decreases the opening of the pelvis.

Additional exercises and positioning suggestions to encourage your baby to get in an optimal position can be found at *www*.*spinningbabies.com*. Keep in mind, every body and every baby is unique, and sometimes the best position for your baby is posterior. If your baby is posterior during labor, these exercises may encourage her to turn. Helping your baby get into an optimal position can contribute to a deeper physical connection to your baby, less pain in labor, and a more positive birth experience.

## Increasing Comfort for You and Your Baby During Labor

It is impossible to know what labor will be like for you and your baby. Therefore, making a final decision now on how you want to cope during labor is premature. What *is* important is to clarify your belief system about your body, your labor, and your perception of pain. Understand that your baby is also physically and emotionally experiencing labor, and your experience in labor will contribute to your baby's experience. Using Conscious Agreement and Conscious Attachment throughout your labor and birth can guide you toward making the best decisions for you and your baby.

### Know Your Options

Explore all of your options for comfort in labor. Prepare yourself with knowledge, surround yourself with the support you need, and make time to practice comfort strategies and relaxation techniques, such as the deep-breathing practices from Chapter 7. This will ensure that no matter how your labor unfolds, you will have the resources you need to cope comfortably and effectively. Preparation and the use of Conscious Agreement and Conscious Attachment is the recipe for a positive birth experience.

This book is not designed as a childbirth manual; however, preparation for your and your baby's comfort in labor starts prenatally. Here are some basic suggestions for you and your partner:

### PRENATAL PERIOD
- Practice Conscious Agreement and Conscious Attachment
- Take a childbirth class that is in alignment with your belief systems
- Read several good books on labor and birth
- Practice comfort strategies with your labor partners
- Strongly consider hiring a labor doula
- Select a place to give birth that feels good to you both
- Visualize your baby
- Connect to your source

### LABOR AND BIRTH PERIOD
- Practice Conscious Agreement and Conscious Attachment
- Labor in a place that feels safe and comfortable
- Nourish and hydrate yourself
- Connect to your support team
- Practice PMA and use positive communication skills
- Rest/nap between contractions, and use movement during contractions
- Use gravity to help your baby move down (change positions often)
- Use the tub and shower for comfort when possible
- Use massage, hot and cold packs, aromatherapy, deep-breathing techniques, or anything else that brings you comfort
- Connect to your source

Please remember that this is only a very basic list of suggestions for comfort. Taking childbirth classes and hiring a doula will introduce you to a wide variety of options to increase your and your baby's comfort during labor and birth.

> **"I think one of the best things we could do would be to help women/parents/families discover their own birth power from within themselves. And to let them know it's always been there, they just needed to tap into it."**
> ~John H. Kennell, World-Renowned Pediatrician
> Specializing in Infant Bonding

## Who Will Be with You During Labor?

Part of creating a safe place during your labor is choosing the people that you want with you, as they will have a significant impact on the way your labor progresses. Decide now who will be with you during your labor. Birth is an exciting event, and your friends and family often want to be a part of it. It's human nature to want to be close to the action. What your well-meaning friends and family do not know is that their mere presence changes the way you will labor. When you feel observed or watched, your labor hormones slow down, which means that your labor slows down too. Some people may even cause you and your baby to become stressed, which will further inhibit your labor and reduce your ability to manage pain and connect to your baby. Labor is biologically designed to be a private, intimate event. When planning your support team, make certain to select only those people in your life you feel the most comfortable around.

Once you've decided who will be invited to attend your labor, the birth, and the days following the birth, make certain you communicate your wishes to everyone who potentially wants to be with you and your baby during this time. You may also want to have a plan in place to deal with uninvited visitors. Keep in mind that your support needs could change while you are in labor. Discuss this with your team now so they allow you the freedom to change your mind when necessary. Your doula or nurse can often offer suggestions if you are concerned about hurting people's feelings. Remember, this is your baby's birth. You have a right to create a sacred space to welcome your baby.

## Communicate Your Labor Wishes

In addition to deciding who will be present for your labor, you will also want to consider communicating your labor wishes to everyone on your team. This includes your partner, your doula, your midwife or OB, and other members of the healthcare team (nurse, midwife's apprentice, etc.). Traditionally, this has been done with a written birth plan, a document you create that spells out your desires during your labor and delivery, including instructions such as "Please only discuss pain medications with me if I ask for them."

Birth plans can be useful tools for:

- Thinking about birthing options prenatally
- Clarifying your belief systems concerning your labor and delivery
- Communicating your wishes to your healthcare team prenatally to promote discussion
- Helping you express your values to everyone on your support team

While birth plans are useful to help clarify your birth vision prenatally, consider the following when thinking about using a birth plan at your labor:

- Sometimes birth plans can create a sense of alienation and distrust between you and your healthcare team. Some mothers write them in an effort to avoid mistreatment at the hospital. They may believe that the hospital and/or the healthcare team they have chosen do not have their best interests at heart. Is this really the environment you want to create? Consider your objectives for writing a birth plan. Is it to communicate your wishes effectively, or is it to protect yourself and your baby from choices not made in Conscious Agreement?

- Healthcare providers often prefer verbal communication versus written instructions. Your and your partner's voices are always more effective communication tools than a written document.

- Birth plans represent what you think you want, given a certain set of circumstances you imagine for your labor and delivery. However, labor is unpredictable and is affected not only by physical circumstances, but also emotional circumstances. Many birth plans leave little room for flexibility.

- Studies show that mothers may experience a sense of failure if their birth does not go according to plan. There is no way to predict the future or know what you and your baby will need until you are in that moment.

What you think about, you bring about. Birth plans are often written out of a place of fear and a desire to control the experience. You cannot control your labor and delivery any more than you can control anything in your future. What you do have control over is how you respond to your circumstances during labor. Here are some effective tools to help you have the birth experience that you want for you and your baby:

- Practice Conscious Attachment at all times throughout labor and birth.

- Use Conscious Agreement during your labor and birth for any and all decisions. This ensures that you are making the best decisions in that moment for you and your baby based on your current circumstances.
- Create a vision board for your labor and delivery instead of a birth plan. Birth plans tend to focus on what you don't want while a vision board shares what you *do* want.
- Have honest conversations with your healthcare providers about what you do and don't want prior to labor to help you and your healthcare team to work together more effectively.
- Carefully select your place of birth and healthcare team early in your pregnancy.

Studies show that positive birth memories are not created by the actual events during the labor and birth, but rather how a mother felt during the birthing process. Empowerment results from conscious preparation and decision-making. Focusing on what you and your baby need and verbally communicating those desires is the best way to manifest a positive birth experience.

## Your Healthcare Team

Throughout pregnancy, labor, and birth, you will be surrounded by healthcare providers who will take care of you and your baby. Conscious Agreement and a personal connection with these individuals will help you feel loved, cared for, and supported, a key element for an attachment pregnancy. Most people spend many hours making selections on new computers or car purchases, but very little time selecting the people who support their health. In fact, the average expectant mother spends less than fifteen minutes selecting a healthcare provider for her pregnancy and will typically select pregnancy care providers based on insurance limitations, convenience of location, or past/current healthcare providers with whom they already have a relationship. Instead of making a snap decision, honor this selection as important to you and your baby for your family's long-term health.

After all, pregnancy is one of the only times in your life that you will seek medical care when you are not sick. Pregnancy is not an illness, so the care that you receive during pregnancy and birth should be empowering and supportive. Seeking providers that support your attachment pregnancy can positively impact your and your baby's entire experience. Your healthcare team includes everyone who will offer support to you throughout pregnancy. If at any time you start to feel that you are not in Conscious Agreement with your healthcare team, it is important to have open communication with them about your concerns, or you may find it necessary to change healthcare providers. Ultimately, you are the one who chooses your support team. If you find that there are major differences in your vision for your birth and your caregiver's practice, then you may want to consider seeking out a new provider with whom you can be in Conscious Agreement.

### Understand Healthcare Providers

Understanding the philosophy and focus of different types of healthcare providers will help you select the appropriate care provider for you and your baby. An obstetrician (physician) is a care provider who specializes in the medical support of pregnancy and childbirth. Though physicians are the most common pregnancy healthcare providers in the United States, another safe option is the midwifery model of care.

The midwife has a practice that focuses on wellness through holistic healthcare management for women throughout their life cycle. If you are considering a home birth, water birth, or unmedicated birth, a midwifery model of care may be your best option. In fact, a midwife may appeal to you even if you plan a hospital birth or want to use medication for pain management. For more information about midwives and how to find them, visit *www.mana.org*.

## Is This Healthcare Provider Right for Me and My Baby?

Part of having an attachment pregnancy is choosing the healthcare providers that support and honor the motherbaby bond. Healthcare providers that view pregnancy and birth as a sacred, holistic experience versus a medical event are more likely to support an attachment pregnancy. Typical characteristics of healthcare providers that would be optimal for an attachment pregnancy include:

- A belief that babies are conscious in utero and influenced by the mother's environment
- A birth philosophy that matches yours
- Supportive of a mother's right to have whomever she wishes at her birth, including a doula
- Low cesarean birth and induction rates (for more information on evidence-based practices see *www.childbirthconnection.org*)
- Comfortable in supporting women in any safe manner in which they choose to labor and give birth (unmedicated or natural childbirth, hypnotherapy, use of tub or shower, position of mother's choice, mobility during labor, epidural)
- Supportive of mothers who wish to have a vaginal birth after cesarean (VBAC)
- Supportive of breastfeeding, skin-to-skin contact, and bonding within the first hour and first days

Although you may not be able to handpick every provider at all times, you do have the responsibility to choose your main healthcare providers wisely and with Conscious Agreement. To determine if you and your baby are in Conscious Agreement with your healthcare provider, start by asking yourself a few questions when you visit with her.

- How do I feel about the care provider's bedside manner?
- Does she smile? Is she warm?

- Do I feel comfortable with her? Do I sense that my baby is at ease during my appointment?
- Does she patiently respond to all of my questions?
- Does she seem well informed and up to date in her thinking?
- Does she ask me how I feel about things?
- Does she seem to be respectful of my time?
- Do I feel cared for by the nurses and other staff at this practice?
- Does she support my desire to have an attachment pregnancy?

Trusting your intuition and asking the right questions is by far the best way to find healthcare providers that will support your attachment pregnancy.

> "All laboring women deserve to be nurtured, loved, attended to, and supported as they undertake the journey to the birth of their child. That journey can be one of the most life changing experiences of their lives. I have always felt that the best answer to this question came from a mother herself when she said to me, 'My doula was my friend, my strength, my shield, my teacher, and, most of all, my anchor in a sea of confusion, pain, and fatigue. She was to me what a lighthouse was to a ship, a gentle guide showing you your destination and helping you avoid unnecessary hazards.'"
>
> ~Polly Perez, Master Doula

### Doula Care

A great addition to the attachment pregnancy team is the labor doula, a nonmedical support professional who is trained to provide physical, emotional, and informational support to the family during pregnancy, labor, and birth. Studies show that the use of a labor doula can improve birth outcomes, increase bonding, increase breastfeeding rates, and enhance overall birth satisfaction. A doula's presence can preserve the sacred space of labor. She can support your choice to practice Conscious Agreement and Conscious Attachment throughout the labor and birth process. Labor doulas can provide a sense of peace and security, which enhances the motherbaby bond during labor, birth, and postpartum. For more information on doulas, visit *www.cappa.net*, *www.dona.org*, or *www.icea.org*.

## Where Will You Have Your Baby?

There are many options for the place of birth, and no single place is right for every mother and baby. The vast majority of women in the United States—well over 90 percent—will give birth in the hospital, although home births and birth center births have recently been on the rise. Each option for birth has advantages and disadvantages, so use careful consideration and Conscious Agreement to make this important decision. Before you consider where you will give birth, take into consideration what place of birth will best support your motherbaby bond. After all, your comfort has a significant impact on how you will labor and birth, and that comfort isn't only related to the physical sensations in labor; it is also about your feelings of safety, support, and overall well-being. Your body is always eavesdropping on your thoughts. This will be true during your labor and birth, thus the importance of feeling safe and supported during the process. Choosing the place where you will give birth is a very personal decision. Not everyone feels comfortable or safe in a hospital, just as not everyone would feel comfortable giving birth at home. This decision is about you and your baby and where you feel safe.

Many families desire the warmth, comfort, and relaxed, family-focused environment that a home birth provides. While hospitals have taken great strides in trying to emulate the look of home, the décor of the hospital has nothing to do with the type of care you will receive there. Do not expect a home birth experience if you plan to give birth in a hospital. Alternatively, do not expect a home birth to offer what a hospital has.

If you have a midwife as your provider, your possible options can include a hospital birth, birth center, or home birth, dependent on how she practices. If you have a physician or obstetrician, it is most likely that she only offers care in a hospital setting. Some obstetricians work in free-standing birth centers alongside midwives, but it is still a rare occurrence in the United States. Often obstetricians will have practicing privileges at several hospital locations, so it is up to you to do your homework to determine which hospital is the best fit for your family if you choose an obstetrician or physician as your provider.

As you make your decision, keep in mind that hospitals are designed to provide medical care for the masses. They are not specifically designed for individualized care or attachment. They have many policies and procedures in place to protect their patients and the hospital staff, which can impact individual freedoms. Hospitals are designed to treat people during illness and emergencies, not necessarily to protect the individual emotional needs and well-being of mothers, babies, and families. It is up to you to be your own advocate at a hospital and surround yourself with a support team who will tend to your emotional needs and support your attachment pregnancy.

### Baby-Friendly Facilities
Breastfeeding is a natural extension of an attachment pregnancy and is the healthiest way to feed and nurture your baby once she is born. In order to optimize your breastfeeding experience, consider choosing a Baby-Friendly facility to give birth in. According to Baby-Friendly USA, "Baby-Friendly facilities have taken special steps to create the best possible environment for successful breastfeeding." These facilities have implemented the Ten Steps to

Successful Breastfeeding that have been recommended by the World Health Organization and UNICEF. To locate a Baby-Friendly facility, visit *www.babyfriendlyusa.org.*

## Mother-Friendly Care

Attachment pregnancy honors the bond between a mother and her baby. In order to honor and protect the motherbaby bond during labor and birth, it is wise to choose a facility that values this experience as well. How you are treated in labor affects your baby physically and emotionally as well as your ability to bond postpartum. The Coalition for Improved Maternity Services sponsors an initiative that is designed to support the philosophical cornerstones of mother-friendly care. These cornerstones include normalcy of the birthing process, empowerment, autonomy, do no harm, and responsibility. To find out more, please visit *www .motherfriendly.org.*

## Create Your Labor Nest

Where you give birth should ultimately be based on where you feel the safest and most comfortable. Whether you choose the hospital, birth center, or your home, it is important that you can create a space, your "nest," that feels safe, private, and as homelike as possible. When you are in your nest, the instinctive part of your brain—where all of your comfort hormones and labor hormones are released—is in control. Your baby is also the most comforted in labor when your feel safe and secure in your nest.

Keep in mind that mammals have the most successful births when they are in an undisturbed atmosphere of privacy and intimacy. For example, have you ever observed a pet in labor? Did you notice that she chose the darkest, quietest, most secluded space she could find to labor in? Animals seek privacy and seclusion when in labor. In fact, it's common that mammals will completely stop their labor if disturbed. Human beings are no exception.

Hospitals frequently encounter women who arrive at the hospital with slowed or stalled contractions, although they had experienced strong and frequent contractions at home. This is due to fact that they had left their "nest" or place of comfort, and the rush to the hospital created worry, anxiety, and stress. These stress hormones reduce the body's ability to labor. Nature is intelligent in its design to protect the baby. If a mother perceives stress and becomes fearful, her body slows labor to protect the baby from being born in a dangerous environment. Unfortunately, many things in our world create a stress response for the human mother, which is why you want to choose a place to labor and birth that feels safe and secure.

When a mother labors, her mammalian brain releases all of the hormones necessary to give birth: oxytocin (the contraction hormone), progesterone (the cervical-softening hormone), and beta-endorphins (comfort hormones). The mammalian brain is known as the instinctive brain and works best when the thinking brain (neocortex) is not being stimulated. Things that activate the thinking brain are:

- Bright lights
- Loud or disruptive noises
- The feeling of being observed or watched
- Unwanted touch or intrusion
- The sense of danger
- Any situation that requires active decision-making

Once the thinking brain is engaged, you are more likely to release stress hormones, such as adrenaline and catecholamines. Stress hormones in early and active labor interfere with the brain's release of oxytocin, which is necessary for a productive labor. All of this means that you need to plan to have your baby in the safest, most comfortable place possible.

### How to Decide?

Where you choose to give birth will affect how you labor and, ultimately, your opportunity to bond in the early hours and days after birth. Do not underestimate the importance of this decision, as it deeply impacts your attachment pregnancy and your attachment to your baby after birth. Here you'll find information that can help you make an informed decision. As you read through the following info, consider the pros and cons and how the idea of laboring at each location makes you feel by practicing Conscious Agreement. Ideally, the place of birth needs to be considered very early on in pregnancy (much earlier than the third trimester). However, if you find at any point that you are no longer in conscious agreement with your previously chosen place of birth, it is within your power to change your mind.

SAFETY

- **Hospital Birth:** Access to immediate emergency services, medications, operating room, and potential access to neonatal intensive care unit.
- **Birth Center:** Close proximity to emergency services, medications, and operating room.
- **Home Birth:** Proximity to emergency services, medications, and an operating room is dependent on the location of the home. Data shows that most home births have low rates of transfers to hospital and lower risk of cesarean section and medical intervention.

COMFORT

- **Hospital Birth:** While you may have access to both medical and nonmedical pain relief, consider that hospitals can limit your ability to move, restrict intake of food, and may not allow use of the tub or shower. Hospitals utilize medical equipment and have policies in place that can interfere with your and your baby's comfort and endorphin release.

- **Birth Center:** You will have access to many natural comfort strategies in a birth center, but there may or may not be access to pain medications. Most birth centers offer continuous labor support, which can contribute to your and your baby's comfort and endorphin release. Many birth centers offer both hydrotherapy and water birth options.
- **Home Birth:** When you are home, you and your baby are in an environment that you have created. You are surrounded by the people, smells, sights, and things that you are most familiar with. You have the freedom to choose the support you want, when and where you want it. You have complete control over your environment, from what you wear to what you eat to who surrounds you. Ask your midwife about access to pain medications, if that is important to you.

ATTENDANTS

- **Hospital Birth:** While you will be able to choose your personal support team, the hospital may restrict the overall number of people supporting you. Children may be discouraged from attending or not be permitted at all. Additionally, you may have very little control over who your healthcare team is, including your doctor.
- **Birth Center:** Most birth centers tend to be more flexible in allowing you to choose your birth team. Check with your local birth center about visitation policies.
- **Home Birth:** You get to choose all of your attendants at your birth. There are no restrictions. Check with your midwife to see who her backup or assistant will be.

NOURISHMENT/HYDRATION

- **Hospital Birth:** Hospitals often have policies that restrict nourishment during labor. This has been shown to have a negative impact on labor and the perception of pain. Use of intravenous fluids (IV) is commonplace in hospitals.

- **Birth Center:** You are encouraged to eat and drink as you wish throughout labor.
- **Home Birth:** Not only can you eat and drink when you wish at home, but you are surrounded by the foods and drinks that you enjoy. You can also have people around you who can cook meals as needed.

### PRIVACY

- **Hospital Birth:** You will have very little privacy at the hospital. You do not get to choose who comes in your room, or even when they come in (with the exception of your own birth team).
- **Birth Center:** While you may have more privacy at a birth center than at a hospital, there still may be times that your privacy is compromised.
- **Home Birth:** It's your home; you decide the level of privacy that you need and have ultimate control over your environment. For example, you may have several friends present in your house during your labor, but you may choose to go to another room.

### MEDICAL PROCEDURES

- **Hospital Birth:** At the hospital, many routine medical policies and procedures are standard, some of which may not be medically necessary and in fact may carry some risk for you and your baby. Familiarize yourself with the routine procedures, and be certain to take a hospital tour and ask questions. By talking to your care provider, you may be able to avoid unnecessary procedures. More than a third of all U.S. women who give birth in a hospital give birth via cesarean section.
- **Birth Center:** Most medical procedures at birth centers are not routine, but are available in the event that they become neces-

sary. Take a tour of your birth center and ask questions about their medical procedures and policies.

- **Home Birth:** The medical procedures that are available at a homebirth are often determined by state laws and by the type of care provider attending the birth. In the event of an emergency or required cesarean, you will need to be transferred to the hospital. The distance between your home and the nearest hospital should be taken into consideration.

### RECORDING YOUR BIRTH

- **Hospital Birth:** Many hospitals have restrictions on still photography, as well as video recording. Check with the hospital and your care provider about their policies.
- **Birth Center:** It is uncommon for birth centers to place restrictions on photography or video recording. However, to be sure, check with your birth center.
- **Home Birth:** You can record anything you wish at a home birth. It is your home and your birth. Check with your midwife to make sure she has no objections.

Your commitment to preparing for your labor and birth during your attachment pregnancy sets the tone for a healthy and peaceful transition for your new family. Taking the time necessary to fully prepare for your baby's birth will help to ensure that the prenatal motherbaby bond you have created will continue to grow.

# CHAPTER SUMMARY

Your physical and emotional preparation for labor and birth will significantly contribute to your and your baby's overall experience. When you are in an environment of safety and security, your body is able to help you and your baby cope with the sensations of labor and birth. The tools that you have perfected during your attachment pregnancy—Conscious Agreement and Conscious Attachment—can guide you toward making the best decisions for you and your baby during labor and birth. Remember:

- Vision boards are graphic collages of images that you personally select to symbolize your wants and needs. They can be used as tools to help you shed light on the things that matter the most to you and your baby and clarify what it is that you really want. A birth vision board is also a great replacement for a traditional birth plan.

- You and your baby will likely have lasting effects from the birth; therefore, thoughtful consideration of your labor and birth options is important for the long-term motherbaby bond.

- How you perceive pain and your experience of the birthing process does impact your ability to further bond with your baby.

- Your ability to feel in control and supported can contribute to a more positive perception of your labor, regardless of the scenario.

- Your positive attitude and perception can help you tap into your intuition and allow you to make the best choices for you and your baby.

- When you have the support you need, you can use the comfort strategies of your choice, and by practicing both Conscious Attachment and Conscious Agreement, you will find that your perception of pain is decreased.

- Maternal movement and positioning affects the way a baby positions herself in the pelvis and can improve the outcome of labor. You can practice optimal fetal positioning to enhance your connection to your baby and help her get in the best position for birth.

- Prepare yourself with knowledge, surround yourself with the support you need, and make time to practice comfort strategies and relaxation techniques.

- Labor is biologically designed to be a private, intimate event. When planning your support team, make certain to select only those people in your life you feel the most comfortable around.

- Birth plans can be an excellent tool for communicating your wants and desires prenatally with your healthcare and support team. However, birth vision boards are better tools for manifesting the birth experience you want.

- Conscious Agreement and a personal connection with your healthcare team will help you feel loved, cared for, and supported during attachment pregnancy and labor and birth.

- Understand the philosophy and focus of the healthcare providers you choose to optimize the care for you and your baby. Healthcare providers that view pregnancy and birth as a sacred, holistic experience versus a medical event are more likely to support an attachment pregnancy.

- Hiring a labor doula can provide a sense of peace and security and can enhance the motherbaby bond during labor, birth, and postpartum.

- Before you consider where you will give birth, take into consideration what place of birth will best support your motherbaby bond. This decision is about you and your baby and where you feel safe.

# CHAPTER 15

# What's Right for Your New Family?

> "The more people have studied different methods of bringing up children, the more they have come to the conclusion that what good mothers and fathers instinctively feel like doing for their babies is the best after all."
>
> ~Benjamin Spock, Pediatrician and Child Advocate

You have been making parenting decisions since the moment you found out you were pregnant. These decisions and your attachment to your baby have influenced the development, health, and personality of your baby. It is now time for you to begin to think about the important decisions and preparation necessary to ease the transition from pregnancy to parenting. The concepts of attachment pregnancy were designed to help you develop a secure relationship with your baby prenatally that inspired confidence in your ability to mother your child. This confidence, combined with preparation for the early parenting period, will be your key to a continued successful motherbaby bond with your newborn.

## You Know What's Right

Undoubtedly, you have already been inundated with both solicited and unsolicited advice about how to raise your baby. Every day you will be faced with parenting decisions, but the most important parenting decision you will ever make is the decision to trust your inner wisdom and listen to your maternal instincts. This can be challenging when the information from influential sources in your life may be in direct conflict with what you believe. This is why it is essential that Conscious Agreement and Conscious Attachment is at the heart of every important decision you make. Your connection to your baby always steers you down the right path.

Your maternal instincts become heightened during pregnancy. In fact, your brain actually changes to make you a better decision-maker as a mother. Your sense of smell, your perception of your environment, and your ability to read the expressions of others become enhanced so that you are better equipped to protect your baby. This is nature's way of protecting the human race. You are designed to be a good mother. Trust yourself.

There are a variety of important decisions that you and your partner must make in the days following birth. These decisions are best made prenatally so that you have the time to weigh all factors and how they will affect your continued motherbaby bond. As with every important decision that you make for yourself and your baby, it is crucial that you are in Conscious Agreement. Remember that the goal is to be in Conscious Agreement with yourself *and* your baby.

As you make the following decisions, keep in mind that the first few days after the birth of your baby are sacred and can have lasting effects on bonding. You will never get these moments back, so make sure to seriously contemplate what you feel is best for your baby during this time.

## Breastfeeding

Though our society tends to view breastfeeding as a choice, it is a biological need for all newborns to receive their mother's milk. Only your milk can provide the immune factors and nutrition that your baby's growing body and brain require. Breastfeeding meets all of the critical needs of your baby: warmth, nourishment, and a loving connection. In fact, the hormones released during breastfeeding are designed to help keep you and your baby in a deep state of attachment. Babies tend to seek out eye-to-eye contact with their mothers while breastfeeding. When you breastfeed, your eyes will dilate from the hormone oxytocin and this sends a message to your baby's brain that she is deeply loved. Additionally, breastfeeding babies automatically receive skin-to-skin contact, which increases oxytocin overall and helps with bonding. Breastfeeding also protects you, the mother, from certain cancers and diseases.

Formula (artificial milk) cannot provide everything that your baby needs, despite what the advertising says. It does not contain the immune factors, enzymes, growth factors, hormones, or antivirals that help to protect, nourish, and develop your baby's body and brain. Without your milk, your baby is at significant increased risk for a variety of diseases like diabetes and allergies.

The decision to breastfeed will have lifelong implications for you and your baby. While the large majority of mothers and babies can successfully breastfeed, there are a few rare situations where families must rely on formula or bottle feeding. Be sure you have exhausted all resources for support and know about all of your options, including donor human milk from milk banks, when making the decision to bottle feed.

### Prepare, Prepare, Prepare

Preparation during pregnancy is essential to breastfeeding success. You can prepare yourself by taking a good breastfeeding class, reading about breastfeeding, going to a breastfeeding support group during pregnancy, planning to use baby-led breastfeeding techniques, and talking with other mothers who have successfully breastfed. Additionally, find out which breastfeeding professionals are in your area to help support you once the baby arrives.

## Skin-to-Skin and Being Near Your Baby

The popularity of hospital nurseries since the 1950s has made it the norm for mothers and babies to be separated periodically in the days following birth. Your baby has a biological need to be close to you, and you and your baby need to be together. When your baby is born, keeping her in direct skin contact actually improves her health. Skin-to-skin contact regulates your baby's metabolism and blood sugar levels. It also helps your baby's brain stay calm, which benefits breastfeeding and overall brain growth. In fact, you might be surprised to learn that your breasts actually change temperature according to your baby's need for warmth.

Research shows that when newborns are separated from their mothers, the baby's brain growth slows down and her stress levels are extremely high. Remember that skin-to-skin also increases the hormone oxytocin, which is the bonding hormone. If you give birth in a hospital that isn't baby-friendly, you may need to advocate for yourself and your baby, because some hospitals may have policies that separate mothers and babies unnecessarily. During your attachment pregnancy you focused on bonding with your baby every day. Don't allow that bond to be compromised in the hospital. You can't bond with your baby from down the hall. Making the conscious decision to stay close to your baby helps you learn how to better care for and bond with your baby.

## Newborn Medical Procedures

Health agencies may require that certain procedures are performed on your newborn baby, depending on the laws in your area. These can include, but are not limited to, procedures such as:

- antibiotic eye ointment
- vitamin K shots
- blood tests
- glucose tests
- hearing tests
- immunizations
- genetic screening

Be aware that many of these procedures can get in the way of early bonding. Sometimes it is possible to delay or refuse these procedures so that early bonding in the first few hours after birth can occur. As a parent, you should educate yourself about the benefits, risks, legal issues, and your rights surrounding these procedures by talking not only to your pediatrician but also to your supportive care providers (such as your doula, childbirth educator, and chiropractor). You can also take a newborn-care class and read good books about newborn care that have an attachment emphasis. In the event that you are not in Conscious Agreement with a certain procedure, you may legally have the right to refuse treatment by signing a waiver. You can talk to your healthcare providers if you have specific questions.

### Circumcision

Circumcision, the surgical removal of the foreskin from the penis, is a decision that some parents of male children will consider. This procedure is sometimes performed for religious or cultural reasons. This decision is often very difficult for parents to make and to agree on. There is no doubt that this is a controversial topic. Due to this controversy, there has been a decade-long trend of reduced circumcision rates. When talking circumcision over with your partner, keep the following facts in mind:

- Circumcision causes pain and physiological stress for the newborn. Circumcision without analgesia is still practiced in the United States in some areas today.
- Physiological responses to circumcision include changes in heart rate, blood pressure, oxygen saturation, and stress levels.
- Circumcised infants exhibit a stronger pain response to subsequent routine immunization than do uncircumcised infants.
- Circumcision can have a negative impact on the baby's ability to breastfeed in the first hours post procedure.

Due to the procedure's physical and emotional impact on a baby boy, this procedure can certainly affect the motherbaby bond, and careful consideration using Conscious Agreement is wise.

## Choosing a Pediatrician or Family Practice Doctor

Selecting a pediatrician or family doctor should be done well before your baby arrives. Your baby's first visit with the pediatrician occurs within a few days of her birth, and the last thing you will have time for in the days following the birth is interviewing and selecting the doctor that is right for your family. The relationship between your family and your doctor could potentially last for up to eighteen years, so careful selection is prudent. You will want to choose a doctor whose values reflect your own family's values and support the concept of attachment parenting. The best way to decide on a provider is to schedule an in-person interview with several doctors, if possible. Pay close attention to how the doctor makes you feel and how he or she answers your questions. It may be helpful to refer to the guide in Chapter 14 on selecting a healthcare provider. Choose your doctor in Conscious Agreement.

## Preparing for Family Attachment

The third trimester is the time to begin to prepare for what life will be like after the birth of your new baby. Making plans early for the arrival of your baby will reduce the amount of chaos you experience in those first few weeks and allow for more family bonding. Many new parents are thrown off-guard by the significant transition that new parenthood brings. The reality of postpartum life is that most of your time will be spent bonding, breastfeeding, sleeping, and eating. There is not much time left over to do anything else, especially entertaining well-meaning friends and family. The info here will help you gather what you need and make decisions ahead of time, which will ultimately lead to less stress for your family. Less stress means a calmer baby, a more peaceful family life, better breastfeeding, more rest, improved bonding for the family, and a faster postpartum recovery.

### Nourishment

You will need to create a plan to nourish your family in the weeks that follow birth. It may seem strange now, but even preparing the smallest meal can seem overwhelming to new moms. If you are not well nourished, then you will not have energy to care for your baby or yourself. Remember the concept of H.A.L.T. and how important it is to try and minimize being hungry, angry, lonely, and tired. Here are some easy ways to prepare to nourish your family:

- Set up meal delivery by friends and family. There are free online programs and apps that can help with organizing meal sign-ups and deliveries. Make certain to communicate that meal delivery should not include a prolonged visit. Be sure to share any dietary restrictions or requests.

- For your baby shower, you can request gift cards to local restaurants that deliver food.
- Ask your partner to create small snack bags or meals for you any time he plans to leave you alone with the baby.
- Make meals ahead of time that can easily be frozen and warmed up when there is no time to cook. In the weeks that precede the birth, when you and your partner make dinner, simply make a double batch and freeze half of it. This is a great date night activity, creating your favorite meals together to share again when the baby is born.

Preparing for your family's nutritional needs ahead of time will significantly improve your early postpartum experience as a new mom.

## Seclusion/Babymoon

Today there are many definitions of the term *babymoon*. However, in terms of an attachment pregnancy, babymoon refers to the intimate family bond. The concept of the babymoon is similar to the idea of a honeymoon. You would not dream of having other people with you on your honeymoon, as it is meant to be a time to get to know one another intimately. Babymooning is meant to be a private, secluded time to get to know the new member of your family in a whole new way. Generally, babymooning means staying in bed, being skin-to-skin with your baby, breastfeeding on cue, eating and drinking when you want, taking lots of naps, and having private time. This means having very limited visitors. You should not have to entertain people while you are recovering from your birth, bonding with your baby, and learning to breastfeed. Make sure you clearly communicate this to your friends and family and tell them that you will let them know when you are ready to accept visitors. You may want to call on friends and family from your sacred circle of support. Ask them to help support your family by dropping off meals, doing errands and light housekeeping, and helping you with your new role.

## Communicate Your Boundaries

Your friends and family will be excited about the new arrival of your baby and often cannot wait to meet her. This means they may drop by unexpectedly or uninvited, which may interrupt precious bonding time. To help avoid these situations you can:

- Leave a note on your door indicating that you are *not* accepting visitors now, but will be accepting visitors at a later time—no exceptions.
- Change the voicemail message on your phone and/or update your social network status. The message should include all of the important information friends and family want to know about your baby, as well as the fact that you are not currently accepting visitors.
- Remember that it is always okay to say no. You can ask that visitors come back at a later time, when invited. You can also share with them that most healthcare providers suggest that babies not be exposed to anyone but the family for the first weeks postpartum.

Proactively communicating your boundaries with your friends and family will help reduce any potential hurt feelings and increase the time available to bond as a new family.

## Housework

Have a discussion with your partner now about housework. It is impossible to care for the baby, yourself, *and* do housework in early weeks of your baby's life. Decide now what critical tasks must be done every day, such as dishes and laundry, and let the rest go. Consider easy ways to get these jobs accomplished.

- Use paper plates and disposable utensils in the first few days.
- Friends and family really want to help, but don't know what to do. Make a list of the things you need done and ask them to pick something to do from your list.
- Ask for money toward a month of maid service at your baby shower. You can also save a few dollars a week throughout your pregnancy for this expense.

Housework should not be a priority in the first few days and weeks after the birth of your baby. Focus instead on bonding time.

### The Ideal Nest

You probably have spent months decorating your nursery. The reality is that most attachment families spend very little time in the nursery. Babies have a biological need to be near their mothers. Make no mistake; a baby monitor does not substitute for your presence. While monitors allow you to hear your baby's cry, crying is a late sign of distress and hunger. The American Academy of Pediatrics recommends that breastfeeding babies sleep in close proximity to their mothers. All babies, whether they are breastfed or bottle fed, benefit from sleeping near their mothers. Keeping your baby near you during sleeping times means that you will want to create a safe space for your baby to sleep. Choose one or two easily accessible rooms that you plan on spending most of your bonding time in, and make sure they are well-stocked with items you and your baby will need (diapers, water, snacks, breast pads, etc.).

*Note:* If you want more information on creating a safe co-sleeping space, look for resources and books from Dr. James McKenna and visit *www.kangaroocareusa.org.*

## Postpartum Help

The following is a list of professionals/groups that can help you in the weeks following the birth. It is helpful to know how to find them before your baby arrives.

- **Lactation Consultants:** These professionals can help you if you experience challenges with breastfeeding. They should have the credential IBCLC, which stands for International Board Certified Lactation Consultant. They can normally be found in hospitals, pediatric offices, or in private practice. You can find a list of IBCLCs at *www.ilca.org.*

- **La Leche League:** This free mother-to-mother support group has been supporting breastfeeding moms since the 1950s. Mothers are encouraged to attend the group meetings even during pregnancy to meet other mothers and become familiar with the league leaders. You can find a list of meetings near you on the La Leche League website at *www.llli.org.* Many hospitals and community centers are now offering breastfeeding support groups as well.

- **Postpartum Doulas:** These doulas specialize in supporting families in the home after the birth. It is important to interview and hire a postpartum doula well before the baby arrives. Often, postpartum doulas are booked well in advance, because they tend to work with only a few families at a time. Postpartum doulas believe in supporting the motherbaby bond and can encourage you to listen to your instincts while providing helpful guidance for the family. You can find postpartum doulas on the CAPPA, DONA, and ICEA websites listed in Chapter 14.

- **New Mother/Breastfeeding Support Groups:** Be aware of the multitude of new mother support groups that are available to you in your area. These can often be found at hospitals, baby stores, WIC (Women Infants Children) offices, churches, libraries, and community centers. There are groups that offer support for different needs, including mothers of multiples, breastfeeding, postpartum depression, back to work, and special needs babies. There are even groups just for dads. Seeking support through community can significantly reduce a new parent's overall stress, provide families with new tools, and extend the family support system. Parents who feel supported tend to have better overall family bonding.

Scouting out the support resources available to you before the baby arrives will make life so much easier by saving you time and energy later on.

## Siblings

Some mothers have fears that they will not be able to love a new baby as much as they love their first child. While your relationship with your new baby will be different, there is no reason to worry that there is not enough love to go around. Love is limitless and there are no boundaries to this emotion. However, don't expect your relationship with the new baby to be the same as the relationship with your first. Every baby is a unique individual and your relationship will develop over time, just as it did with your first child. If you are concerned about this, it may be comforting to talk to mothers who have more than one child about their experiences. Just as you will develop a new relationship with your baby, her sibling(s) will also need time to make the transition. While exciting, becoming a big brother or sister can be overwhelming for some children. Following are some suggestions to help make this transition easier and support a healthy bond between the older children and the new baby.

### Include Your Older Child
Include your older child in the practice of Conscious Attachment when you can. Encourage your child to talk to the baby during the pregnancy. Let your child know that the baby is getting to know him or her already, even though she is still inside of mommy. Helping your child to get to know the new baby prenatally will help to strengthen their sibling relationship once the baby arrives.

### Celebrate!
Celebrate your child's new role in becoming a big brother or sister. Having a new baby is also a rite of passage for your child. Small gestures can go a long way toward making your child feel more included and important in the new role as big brother or sister. You and your partner can research and decide on some specific ways you can honor this new role for your child. For example, some families have a special big brother or sister party before the birth to celebrate this special transition and new role for their child.

### Let Your Child Be Present
Have your children attend the birth of their new brother or sister. It can be a meaningful experience for everyone. If your child wants to be present and you are comfortable having him at the birth, you should prepare him for what he might see and hear in advance. It can be scary for your child to see you in pain or hear you make unfamiliar noises. Keep in mind that you and your partner will not have the capacity at some points in labor to comfort and care for his needs. This means that all young children present at birth should have their own support person to care for them. Careful preparation ahead of time can make the birth of the new baby a joyful experience for the entire family.

### Take a Class

Find a sibling class to teach your child how to safely interact with the new baby. These classes are designed to make your child feel special while also helping to set up safe boundaries for interacting with his or her new brother or sister. Additionally, you can find many movies and books on becoming a big brother or sister at your local library or on the Internet.

### Spend One-On-One Time

After the baby arrives, make sure to plan special time with your older child. Make a conscious effort to create one-on-one time with your older child every day. While you and your partner may find that you may initially have limited opportunities to do this, you can ask other family members and friends to step in and give your child extra love and attention. Try and set up short play dates for your child as often as possible after the baby arrives.

### Make Breastfeeding Time Special

Make breastfeeding a special time for everyone. You can make breastfeeding "family time" by planning activities for your older child in advance. An example of this might include offering special snacks, books, or toys that are only brought out while you are breastfeeding. Keep in mind that some previously weaned toddlers may display a renewed interest in breastfeeding. This is normal and natural behavior and something to consider before the baby arrives.

## Let's Talk about Sex

A baby changes your entire life. Your body will change. Your time and energy resources will change. Your relationship with your partner will change. These changes bring both challenges and opportunities for your relationship. You will need to find new definitions for intimacy. Generally, during the first six weeks postpartum, sexual intercourse is not recommended because your body is healing from the birth process. However, intimacy is well advised. Cuddling, hugging, kissing, and snuggling all can help you and your partner stay connected and contribute to the family bond.

It's also important to realize that your hormones will make a huge shift post pregnancy. These hormonal changes can cause vaginal dryness, decreased sex drive, and breast tenderness. Additionally, many women experience soreness and swelling in the perineum and vaginal area. Some women may also be recovering from a cesarean section, a perineal tear, or an episiotomy. This can make the thought of having sex again a little frightening. Careful planning before resuming sexual intercourse can make the experience less stressful and more enjoyable. Be sure you plan for enough time and privacy, and make sure you have any products you might need, such as lubricant.

Have open and honest conversations with your partner about your feelings regarding sex and intimacy. Don't assume that your partner understands what your body is going through, or that you understand his needs either. Communication is key to the health of your relationship and the overall bond of your family. Men feel most bonded to their partners when they have a satisfying sex life with them. Both partners have needs that are important. If you ignore one another's needs, it becomes more and more difficult as time passes to maintain a healthy relationship. Discuss ways that you both can have your intimacy needs met, even when you may be tired and time is tight. Be creative; intimacy isn't just sex.

## Attachment Parenting

At no other time during life can humans possibly be more attached than during pregnancy. During this period of primal attachment, you and your baby are in absolute physical and emotional connection. This extraordinary period of development literally creates the motherbaby bond you now know. Attachment pregnancy and parenting starts on an emotional level the moment you become mindful of your baby as a person. Once this occurs, your deepest desires are to provide protection, love, and security for your baby. Thus, the concept of attachment parenting is something many mothers will experience biologically as an extension of an attachment pregnancy.

Attachment parenting is a philosophy that was originally coined by pediatrician William Sears. This philosophy is based on the early research on attachment theory by John Bowlby, who found that healthy human emotional development requires a newborn to develop a secure and loving attachment to her care providers. In order for attachment to occur, babies need to bond with their care providers (parents) from birth. This theory has been refined over the past sixty years to focus on a lifestyle that begins in pregnancy and continues throughout the child's life. This style of parenting is grounded in the knowledge that babies have an intrinsic need to be nurtured and loved in a very real physical and emotional way.

Attachment parenting families often include the following practices: breastfeeding (or compassionate baby-led bottle feeding), sleeping in close proximity to the children, offering plenty of loving touch to their children (skin-to-skin, infant massage, babywearing, hugs and kisses, etc.), and practicing a positive, nonviolent discipline approach. Attachment parenting is not necessarily a method that must be followed rigorously. It is a style of parenting that involves the B-O-N-D: Be-ing, observing, nourishing, and deciding based on the needs of your baby and your family. Every family's style of attachment parenting will look different because every family and every baby is unique. Staying in Conscious Agreement can help your family stay truly "attached" at all times. Learn more about attachment parenting at the website for Attachment Parenting International at *www.attachmentparenting.org*.

# Congratulations!

The decisions that you make now will forever shape your child's life and the direction of your family. It is a huge responsibility to become a parent, and the decisions of parenting should not be taken lightly. However, when you stay in a space of consciousness and love when making decisions, you will be guided toward your parenting destiny. Trusting yourself is a skill that you will learn over time as a parent. There will be times when you may make mistakes and you will learn from them. This is what will help build your confidence to make better decisions going forward and trust your intuition. These experiences will make you a better decision-maker, a better parent. This is part of the process of learning to forgive yourself for the mistakes that you make along the path of life and correct your drift. Equally important is allowing yourself to celebrate your successful decisions. It is important for your children to watch these moments of personal forgiveness, celebration, and growth.

While you may have come to the end of this book, you are really at a beginning. It's the beginning of a new you, a new family, and one of the most profound relationships you will ever have. Becoming a mother is a journey that will bring you the greatest love you will ever experience, while also experiencing incredible joy, pain, and sorrow. Your children will present you with the lessons of a lifetime. They will teach you patience and compassion and will push you to the very edge of sanity. All the while, you will be astonished by the very depth of your love for them. You will learn that you are stronger than you ever knew you could be. There will be mistakes made along the journey. Life is messy; it's juicy, it's joyful, it's terrifying, and it's supposed to be that way. Out of the chaos comes beauty, and this is the lesson of mothering.

While this book has given you guidance to help you through your attachment pregnancy, hopefully you remember that you already have all of the answers inside yourself. You have every parenting answer you will ever need. When you need answers, remember

Conscious Agreement, listen carefully to your inner wisdom, and trust yourself. You are about to meet the love of your life. We wish you love, laughter, joy, and strength along your journey. Ultimately, we wish you and your baby the deepest bond and love you will ever know: that of the motherbaby bond.

> **"When someone makes a decision, he is really diving into a strong current that will carry him to places that he had never dreamed of when he first made the decision."**
>
> ~Paulo Coelho, Author of *The Alchemist*

# CHAPTER SUMMARY

The most important parenting decision you will ever make is the decision to trust your inner wisdom and listen to your maternal instincts. The decisions surrounding pregnancy, labor, birth, and early parenting affect the future emotional and physical health of your entire family. Remember:

- Breastfeeding meets all of the critical needs of your baby: warmth, nourishment, and a loving connection.

- Your baby has a biological need to be close to you. When your baby is born, keeping her in direct skin contact actually improves her health.

- Educate yourself about the benefits, risks, legal issues, and your rights surrounding medical procedures performed on newborns, because many of these procedures can get in the way of early bonding.

- The physical and emotional stress of circumcision affects the motherbaby bond, and careful consideration using Conscious Agreement is wise.

- Choose a doctor whose values reflect your own family's values and support the concept of attachment parenting.

- Making plans early for the arrival of your baby will reduce the amount of chaos you experience in those first few weeks and allow for more family bonding.

- Create a plan to nourish your family in the weeks that follow birth.

- Practice "babymooning" by staying in bed, being skin-to-skin with your baby, breastfeeding on cue, eating and drinking when you want, taking lots of naps, and having private time.

- Develop a strategy to communicate your boundaries with friends and family that will ensure your privacy and protect your bonding postpartum.

- Decide now what critical tasks must be done every day, such as dishes and laundry, and let the rest go.

- All babies, whether they are breastfed or bottle fed, benefit from sleeping near their mothers.

- Create a list of professionals/groups/resources that can help you in the weeks following the birth.

- Have a plan in place if you have other children to make the transition with a new baby at home easier and to support a healthy bond between the older children and the new baby.

- During the first six weeks postpartum, sexual intercourse is not recommended, so you will need to find new definitions for intimacy for a short time.

- Attachment parenting is a style of parenting that involves the B-O-N-D: Be-ing, observing, nourishing, and deciding based on the needs of your baby and your family. It can include breastfeeding (or compassionate baby-led bottle feeding), sleeping in close proximity to the children, offering plenty of loving touch to the children (skin-to-skin, infant massage, babywearing, hugs and kisses, etc.), and practicing a positive, nonviolent discipline approach.

# Notes from the Authors

We would like to thank you for reading *The Attachment Pregnancy*. Both of us have experienced very unique journeys along the path to writing this book. We hope the following will give you some insight as to why the concepts in this book are so important for us to share with you.

## From Tracy Wilson Peters

My journey to become a pregnancy and childbirth expert really started with my first pregnancy, when I was just eighteen years old. At that time, I knew nothing about pregnancy, birth, or babies. The one thing I did know was that I wanted to be a good mother and give my child a good life, filled with love. I received a necklace that said "#1 Mom," and it was my most treasured possession. I think that even then at eighteen years old, I somehow knew that what we think about, we bring about.

Despite wanting to be a great mother, I certainly made my share of mistakes along the way. I have always said that my son Hunter and I really grew up together. Even though I became a mother at such a young age, I have thankfully managed to raise two incredible sons, Hunter and Foster (eight years apart), who have both grown up to be loving, intelligent, and compassionate people.

What would I do differently? Don't we all occasionally wish we had a time machine so that we could go back and do things a little bit differently? There are a few things I do wish I could go back and change; wishing my pregnancy would go by faster, not treasuring every single movement I felt my babies make inside me, not reading just one more book at bedtime when asked, and working so many hours. These are all typical mommy regrets. The thing I wish I could change the most, though, is what I did not know at the time. When Laurel and I began our research on this topic, I was astounded to learn how very conscious and aware babies are in utero. During our research, I remember seeing a baby crying in utero on ultrasound and from that moment on, I never thought of pregnancy or babies the same way again. My work as a pregnancy expert became even more important to me than it had ever been before. I wish that I had known then about the consciousness of our babies (even in utero) and how much they are absorbing from us from the moment their lives begin. None of us can go back and change our past, and none of us are responsible for what we did not know at the time.

I want you to know that you have the power to shape a human being's life. You have the power to change your child's world and make it a better place by the choices that you make in each and every moment. Your choices affect your baby, they affect you as a woman, and they affect your family. Everything you do matters. In every mundane moment there are hidden opportunities to create love in your life. These opportunities begin in your consciousness. The opportunity to create love is always available in the present moment and comes from your own self-awareness. The information is this book can be transformational; it can change pregnancy from a burden to endure into a sacred time of bonding and attachment to cherish. When a mother learns that she can experience a deep connection to her baby during pregnancy, and that her baby is already depending on her for security, it can change her whole view of pregnancy. The human race needs hope; we need a global shift in consciousness, and we need to value each other and remember that we are all connected. During pregnancy, every mother on the planet has the opportunity to shape a human being, the opportunity to literally change the future. When a baby experiences love through an attachment pregnancy, that baby is born in love. Shouldn't we all be born in love?

## From Laurel Wilson

This continued project, from the first edition of *The Greatest Pregnancy Ever* to this edition of *The Attachment Pregnancy*, has been the manifestation of a long-held wish. Since the very first quickening in my belly with my first child, I knew with every cell of my body that my child was connected to me beyond the umbilical cord. I intuitively felt that my world was shaping his world, and I desired to create a world into which this child would feel welcomed. I was very young, scared, and not ready to be a mother. The early weeks of pregnancy were a roller coaster of emotions. I struggled between feeling a deep bond with the child growing inside me, and a sense of panic that somehow I would do the wrong thing, eat the wrong food, or do something to cause irreparable harm to my baby. I was functioning in a heightened state of anxiety and fear, which stemmed from only wanting and wishing for the best for my baby.

At that time, I did not know that wanting and loving my child would have the most significant impact on the healthy development of my child, or that my state of mind would lay the foundation for who he would become. I did not know that addressing my fears would have been better than all of the coffee I passed by, all of the fresh fruit I ate, and all of the stretching and swimming I did to have a healthy pregnancy. Even though I was not aware of the importance of stress reduction and dealing with my fears, I did intuitively know that forming a relationship with my child did not start at his birth. It was happening every moment during my pregnancy, with the division of every cell, with every flutter of his limbs, and with every thought I had. The challenging moments of his birth and what followed were eased by the knowledge that this little person already knew me and was grounded in the depth of my love for him.

With my next pregnancy, my awareness of the motherbaby bond deepened. Though my stress levels and fears increased, I still knew that what mattered most was my relationship to this child. My pregnancies, births, and breastfeeding experiences with my sons, Trevor and Ryan, led me on my path of discovery as a childbirth and breastfeeding professional. At first it was a means of healing myself, and later it became a means of spiritual awakening and service to my community. This work has challenged and rewarded me nearly every day. It has led me to a greater awareness of the emotional life of the mother and child, and it has deepened my respect for life and the universal laws that support this life I live.

Unfortunately, our society tends to value things that are truly inconsequential in the great scope of humanity. We are a society that honors hard work, money, the acquisition of material objects, and the ability to multitask. While these values are not "bad," they allow us to misdirect our attention, changing focus from what really matters to the human being to the ideals of the ego. French Jesuit and philosopher Pierre Teilhard de Chardin said, "We are not human beings on a spiritual journey. We are spiritual beings on a human journey." Today there is a lack of human connection during pregnancy; a societal lack of honoring this sacred and integral period. How we come into existence matters. How we are conceived, what our parents think, and how our parents love themselves and one another matters.

Merriam-Webster defines consciousness as "the quality or state of being aware, especially of something within oneself." Our culture is in a state of unconsciousness; our internal awareness is dulled. We no longer trust our instincts for pregnancy and motherhood. Families seek 4-D ultrasound, consult with machines and lab tests, and compare their own experience with strangers on television. The beautiful stillness of our beginnings has been lost; the peacefulness that invites a woman to place a hand over her belly and know, really know in every cell in her body, that this being inside her is beauty personified has somehow been lost in the shuffle.

The exquisite beauty of parenthood is the story being told with each and every pregnancy and birth and in every moment that a baby finds her entire world at her mother's breast. We have the ability and the responsibility to create peace in these moments. I wish to share the information in this book so that a shift can take place in our societal expectations of pregnancy and mothering. I wish for you to experience how spirit and science combine to make us who we are through an attachment pregnancy.

# Acknowledgments

Words cannot express how much it meant to us to have Robin Grille write our foreword and to have his continued support of our mission involving attachment pregnancy. Polly Perez, we thank you for sharing your knowledge with us and believing in our message. Tammy Archer, thank you for being our original test mom and helping us stay on the right path. We owe a debt of gratitude to both Barbara Decker and Lisa Reagan for their enthusiasm and support during this journey. The CAPPA Dream Team and faculty deserve specific recognition for their ability to embrace and share the concepts in our book with open hearts. Natalie, Mandy, JoAnna, and Lisa, we are so thankful for all of the important things you did, without which we could not have finished our project on time. We want to thank Steve Harris for believing in our message and seeking the right home for our project. Finally, we wish to thank the team at Adams Media for their guidance and assistance in publishing our work.

**From Laurel:** This book grew out of a grateful heart and love that is unceasing and ever expanding for my family: my sons Trevor and Ryan, my husband Dan, my brother Harley and his family, and our parents Jane, Don, Patricia, and Marvin. The constant love you all have given me has inspired me to be better person, a better advocate, a better mother, a better wife, and a better daughter. Trevor, your birth proved to me that even profound birth trauma can be healed with love and gave me the personal knowledge for the foundation of this book. Ryan, your smiles from the moment of your birth further proved to me that a happy momma makes a happy baby. Thank you, Danny, for your absolute belief in me. You are my sequoia, able to stand strong, bend, and protect us all when I become a hurricane. The depth of my love for you has not yet been located. Thank you, Mom and Dad. Growing up, I never once doubted that love existed in every molecule of the universe because I was so thoroughly loved by you both. Terry, you opened my mind to concepts that unnerved and excited me. Thank you for your love and for teaching me that consciousness is what it's all about. Fred Wirth, I send my gratitude to the great unknown for teaching me that babies are conscious and seeking love from conception. You changed the course of my professional life. Robin Sales, I am so grateful that you offered me the opportunity to heal my broken heart through prenatal yoga. Trish, for listening to me chatter endlessly about babies and mommas and still picking up the phone every time I ring, I love you. Karen, you are my touchstone. Thank you for helping me live what I preach. To the extraordinary women in my life, thank you for helping me grow into the woman who could write this book. Finally, thank you, Tracy. With you at my side, with your unwavering belief in what we are doing, we will see the world change one momma and baby at a time. Thank you for your love, and even more, thank you for your faith in our concept. I am so proud of the woman you are and your willingness to be open to new ideas, even when they are terrifying. Together the possibilities are endless.

**From Tracy:** I want to first acknowledge my husband, Mark, and my sons, Hunter and Foster. The love and support that you all give me is why I was able to accomplish writing this book. Thank you for your sacrifices along the way. Thank you to my parents and sisters for loving me and for your support. Polly Perez has been a mentor and a friend to me, showing me love and support throughout my career. Polly inspires me to never give up on a dream. I'd like to thank Janice and Barry Banther for their friendship, love, and good advice over the years. I'd like to thank the entire leadership team at CAPPA; you are all so special to me and I am so grateful for your love and confidence. I'd like to thank the staff at the CAPPA office for always being available to give me opinions and support and for correcting my typos. Last but not least, Laurel. People sometimes see that our last names are the same and assume that we are sisters. I've been asked that often since we started writing the book together. I want you to know, Laurel, that you are my sister. You are such a loving person and you have enlightened me to so many things since we began working together. Thank you for helping me make the shift. I don't feel like the same person I was when we began this book, and I know that you are not either. We have grown together, learned together, and laughed together. I can never thank you enough for your friendship, your heart, and for making me swim with stingrays (literally and figuratively).

# Index

# About the Authors

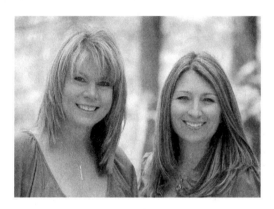

**Laurel Wilson, IBCLC, CCCE, CLD, CLE,** has more than two decades of experience working with families and professionals as a childbirth and lactation educator/trainer/consultant, doula, and prenatal yoga instructor. Laurel takes a creative approach to working with the pregnant family, helping families to connect with their inner resources to discover their true beliefs about themselves, their relationships, and their abilities to birth and parent their children. Laurel has successfully trained hundreds of professionals to become childbirth and lactation educators, labor doulas, and prenatal yoga teachers. She has been featured as a pregnancy and breastfeeding expert in professional videos and webinars. Laurel has been joyfully married to her husband for more than twenty years and has two beautiful sons, whose difficult births led her on a path toward helping emerging families create positive experiences. She believes that the journey into parenthood is a life-changing rite of passage that should be deeply honored and celebrated.

**Tracy Wilson Peters, CCCE, CLD, CLE,** has been a lifelong advocate for families and babies. Married for over two decades and mother to two amazing sons, Tracy's experience raising her own children led her to a love for supporting expectant families. This passion encouraged her to found CAPPA, Childbirth and Postpartum Professionals Association. Tracy serves as both the CEO and as a faculty member for CAPPA, the largest childbirth education organization in the world. Internationally known as a pregnancy expert, she has authored numerous articles and appeared on many television networks, including FOX, CBS, and NBC. Tracy has worked with expectant women and families for nearly two decades, attending hundreds of births as a professional labor doula and teaching classes to more than 3,000 families.

For inquiries on speaking engagements, lectures, and book signings, please e-mail Tracy and Laurel at *info@attachmentpregnancy .com*. For more information on the concepts in this book, current research, and resources visit *www.theattachmentpregnancy.com*.